Parkinson's Dise
Dummies®

By
Michele Tagliati, MD
Gary N. Guten, MD, MA
Jo Horne, MA

Volume 1 of 2

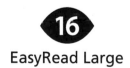

16

EasyRead Large

RHYW

Copyright Page from the Original Book

TABLE OF CONTENTS

Foreword by Deborah W. Brooks
President and CEO of The Michael J. Fox Foundation
for Parkinson's Research

About the Authors

Michele Tagliati, MD, is a movement disorders specialist with extensive experience in the diagnosis and treatment of Parkinson's disease. As Director of the Parkinson's Disease Center at Mount Sinai Medical Center in New York, he follows hundreds of patients at several stages of disease progression. He dedicates his professional life to caring for PD patients and developing research protocols that will ultimately improve their condition. In particular, Dr. Tagliati is a leader in the field of deep brain stimulation for PD and dystonia. He currently serves as teaching faculty at the annual courses given on DBS programming at the American Academy of Neurology and the International Movement Disorders Society. He has published over 40 peer-reviewed articles and 20 book chapters. A medical graduate and neurologist specialist from the University of Rome in Italy, he moved to New York in 1991 with a PD research scholarship. After completing a second neurology residency at Mount Sinai Medical Center, Dr. Tagliati served as a faculty member at Albert Einstein College of Medicine and then moved back to Mount Sinai to become Division Chief of Movement Disorders. He is currently Associate Professor of Neurology at Mount Sinai School of Medicine and a diplomate of the American Board of Psychiatry and Neurology.

Gary N. Guten, MD, MA, is qualified to contribute to this book for three reasons: He's a sports medicine orthopedic surgeon, author, and Parkinson's patient. As an orthopedic surgeon, he specializes in sports medicine, exercise, and nutrition. He was the founder of Sports Medicine and Orthopedic Center in Milwaukee, Wisconsin. The center now has eight doctors. As an author, he has published six books on sports medicine and 27 medical journal publications—14 are on the Web site of the National Library of Medicine accessible at www.pubmed.com. As a Parkinson's patient, his insight and understanding of Parkinson's disease comes from the fact that he developed PD in 1995. He had to stop doing surgery—but continues to actively do office practice and consultations. Gary received his medical degree from the University of Wisconsin, and as a lifelong learner received a Master of Arts degree in 2005 in Bioethics from the Medical College of Wisconsin. His master's thesis subject was *Placebo Surgery* with a critical analysis of stem cell surgery for PD.

Jo Horne, MA. Many factors came together to lead Jo to this project. After receiving her master's degree in communications from the University of Cincinnati, she spent the early years of her career as a college lecturer. Later as she began an eight-year journey as the long-distance caregiver for her parents, she became aware of the need for a comprehensive guide for caregivers. Over the next several years she wrote three such guides, all published by AARP. At the same time, she left teaching to work with her husband as he and others pioneered the concept of adult day care in the state of Wisconsin. She was also a fellow of the Midwest Geriatric Education Center's initial class and was tapped to deliver the keynote address at the national meeting of the Association of University Professionals in Health Administration for her work in developing curriculum on professional/patient interactions in long-term care. Her work as a communications manager in the dual corporate worlds of long-term care insurance and later the pharmaceutical industry further prepared her to research and write on the effects of Parkinson's on patients and their care partners. Finally when her sister was diagnosed with PD, Jo found herself up close and personal with the impact PD can have. Her unique combination of personal and professional experience has made her a popular speaker and workshop leader as well as a guest expert for national television and radio talk shows.

Dedication

Michele Tagliati, MD—In memory of my father, Silvano Tagliati, who suffered with great dignity from Parkinson's disease, and my beloved wife, Tracy, who greatly inspired my life as a man and a doctor.

Gary N. Guten, MD, MA—This book is dedicated to the lasting memory of my neurologist, Dr. Steven Park, who died in 2006 from a tragic accident. Not only was he a Parkinson's disease maven, but he was my medical mentor, respected colleague, and golfing buddy.

Jo Horne, MA—Every book is for Larry, whose belief in me has never wavered. This one is also especially for Patsy Horne DeBord—my sister and friend—whose fight with PD brought our family closer in spite of the years and miles separating us. It is also for my siblings, Betsy and Earle, and in-laws, Tom and Carole, who took on the demanding role of care partner for Patsy without hesitation and—learning on the job—performed it with love.

Authors' Acknowledgments

Michele Tagliati, MD—I would like to thank Jo, whose enlightened spirit envisioned and inspired this book, and all my patients, who teach me a great deal about their disease every day. In addition, I would like to thank the Department of Neurology at Mount Sinai Medical Center and the Bachmann-Strauss Dystonia & Parkinson Foundation for their continuous support.

Gary N. Guten, MD, MA—One person stands out as being responsible for my insight, knowledge, and fight against Parkinson's disease. That person is my piano teacher—Rita Shur. She has taught me to play the piano (or write)—not with my fingers—but with my heart and my head.

Jo Horne, MA—Without the unique expertise and indefatigable dedication of Michele and Gary, this project would still be on the drawing board. I am indebted to both of them for their insights and humor as we made this journey. I am also deeply indebted to my agent Natasha Kern and everyone on the project team at Wiley Publishing. But as Willie Loman said in the Arthur Miller play *Death of a Salesman,* "Attention must (also) be paid" to the dozens of PWP, their care partners, and healthcare professionals who contributed to the work just by showing me what it means to live with PD. Finally I am profoundly indebted to those fearless and tireless warriors at the foundations and organizations who daily wage the battle to find a cure. My deepest wish is that they make this book obsolete in a very short time.

Publisher's Acknowledgments

We're proud of this book; please send us your comments through our Dummies online registration form located at www.dummies.com/register/.

Some of the people who helped bring this book to market include the following:

Acquisitions, Editorial, and Media Development

Senior Project Editor: Alissa Schwipps

Acquisitions Editor: Michael Lewis

Copy Editor: Pam Ruble

Technical Editor: Ramón Luis Rodríguez, MD

Senior Editorial Manager: Jennifer Ehrlich

Editorial Assistants: Erin Calligan, Joe Niesen, David Lutton

Cover Photo: © Stockbyte

Cartoons: Rich Tennant (www.the5thwave.com)

Composition Services

Project Coordinator: Jennifer Theriot

Layout and Graphics: Lavonne Cook, Denny Hager, Stephanie D. Jumper, Barry Offringa, Alicia B. South, Erin Zeltner

Special Art: Kathryn Born, Medical Illustrator

Anniversary Logo Design: Richard Pacifico

Proofreaders: Jessica Kramer, Techbooks

Indexer: Techbooks

***

Publishing and Editorial for Consumer Dummies

Diane Graves Steele, Vice President and Publisher, Consumer Dummies

Joyce Pepple, Acquisitions Director, Consumer Dummies

Kristin A. Cocks, Product Development Director, Consumer Dummies

Michael Spring, Vice President and Publisher, Travel

Kelly Regan, Editorial Director, Travel

Publishing for Technology Dummies

Andy Cummings, Vice President and Publisher, Dummies Technology/General User

Composition Services

Gerry Fahey, Vice President of Production Services

Debbie Stailey, Director of Composition Services

Foreword

A diagnosis of Parkinson's disease is a life-altering event. There is no one way to deal with it. Everyone has a unique set of circumstances, and every patient experiences Parkinson's differently. That's why one book on PD can never be all things to all people. Whether you are living with the disease or are a caregiver or friend to someone who is, you will come to rely on a wide variety of high-quality books, manuals, Web sites, resources and tools. You may be surprised by the voracity of your appetite for newer, better, and just plain more information about PD. And since Parkinson's is—for now, at least—a disease that stays with you for life, your information needs may evolve and change over time.

This book represents something incredibly important: a place to start. We commend its emphasis on tenets that we at The Michael J. Fox Foundation strive to incorporate into our work: an action orientation, a problem-solving mentality, and the distillation of a great deal of complicated information into clear, logical next steps.

Most importantly, the Foundation shares with the authors of this book a commitment to keep patients front and center in every decision we make. As the largest funder of Parkinson's research outside the federal government, we actively partner with scientists to innovate new funding mechanisms that can maximize the quality, quantity and pace of PD research. With a comprehensive view of the field and proactive management of the grants in our portfolio, we are ideally positioned to bridge the gap between basic research and the clinic. For years scientists have asserted that with sufficient research funding, a cure for Parkinson's is within reach. We are working urgently to prove them right.

I am continually inspired by the patients I meet who are endeavoring to live their lives beyond the potentially limiting effects of this disease, defining themselves by their achievements, not their struggle with PD. But no one who knows Parkinson's would suggest that a positive outlook is achievable all the time. Do everything you can to put the odds on your side: Find doctors you trust and can build relationships with; eat well and exercise as much as possible; appreciate and invest in your family and friendships; investigate ways to reduce stress and practice what works for you.

And know that work is continuing aggressively to make this disease, finally, a thing of the past.

Debi Brooks

President and CEO, The Michael J. Fox Foundation for Parkinson's Research

Introduction

If the very idea of a Parkinson's disease diagnosis scares the bejeebers out of you, take a deep breath and pay attention. Although Parkinson's is a chronic and progressive condition with no cure (yet), the strides made in just the last decade to control and manage symptoms are impressive and hopeful. Also the number of national organizations (not to mention big-name celebrities) that are placing the spotlight squarely on the need for a cure is unparalleled.

And we're here to help: An experienced neurologist and lecturer on the treatment of Parkinson's disease (PD); another physician—not a neurologist but rather one who has been living with his own PD (and finding new and innovative ways to maintain control over his life) for over a decade; and a writer of books on aging and giving care whose oldest sister has PD. Together we give you the facts you need, resources you can rely on, and tips on how best to structure your life so that—to paraphrase the popular slogan—you have PD, but it doesn't have you.

This book is your guide to understanding and living with PD. While you—the person with Parkinson's (PWP) are the primary audience—feel free to share *Parkinson's Disease For Dummies* with family, friends, and especially that person who will most likely make this journey with you—your care partner.

We—the doctor-athlete who's fought PD for over ten years, the writer who's seen dozens of people triumph over their PD, and the neurologist who's not in the business of giving up—wish you the strength to persevere, the will to keep fighting for a cure, and the physical and emotional stamina for a long, productive life.

About This Book

At first glance the idea of a *For Dummies* guide to Parkinson's disease may seem ludicrous or even downright insulting. But those of you who have used these guides understand that the dummies reference indicates a guide that presents its topic in simple, straightforward terms. Although PD doesn't have a cure, it can be well managed for years before a person faces its more challenging aspects. And that's what this guide is about—practical ways you can control and manage the symptoms of your Parkinson's so you can get on with your life!

Now, this is not some sugar-coated Pollyanna guide to living with PD. It's a realistic look at what you're facing. It provides solid information and resources to help you and your family come to terms with PD as a factor in all your lives. It offers proven techniques and tips to help you prepare for the future without projecting the worst. And most of all, it reminds you that living a full and satisfying life—in spite of PD—is definitely possible, even probable.

We designed each chapter of *Parkinson's Disease For Dummies* to be self-contained so that you don't have to read the book sequentially or read the first parts to understand any later chapters. You can dip in and out wherever you please and concentrate only on what you need. The table of contents and the index can help guide your search.

Conventions Used in This Book

The following conventions are used throughout the text to make the info consistent and easy to understand:

- New terms appear in *italic* and are closely followed by an easy-to-understand definition. We also clearly define the terms in the handy glossary at the back of the book.

- **Bold** is used to highlight the action parts of numbered steps.

This guide has a few special conventions that are widely accepted by Parkinson's researchers and advocates as well as by people with PD and their families:

- Parkinson's disease is often abbreviated *PD.*

- A person diagnosed and living with PD is often re-ferred to as *PWP,* or person (or persons) with Parkinson's.

- Because PWP are fully capable of making decisions and planning their care for many years following diagnosis, we refer to their primary care-givers as *care partners.* There may come a day when you need more hands-on care and assistance. Should that day come, that's when your *care partner* takes on the additional role of *caregiver.*

- Although we hope your family and close friends will read many portions of this guide, some sec-tions are do-not-miss for these folks. Several chapters have a section titled "A Word for the PD Care Partner" at the end. Be sure to share these sections with the person (or persons) most likely to be your support and eventual caregiver.

Foolish Assumptions

In putting together this guide to living with PD, the three of us have assumed the following about you:

- That you have (or suspect you have) PD yourself or are close to someone who does.

- That you want reliable information about PD, and you're looking for proven ways (techniques and resources) to treat and manage its symptoms.

- That you intend to take a proactive role in facing this challenge and not simply (blindly!) do everything the first healthcare provider you see tells you to do.

- That you're open to lifestyle adjustments and complementary or alternative techniques that are proven to manage symptoms and prolong functions.

- That you realize PD is not just a physical condition that affects only you; it has elements that impact you—and everyone who cares about you—physically, mentally, and emotionally. You all need to be proactive in preparing for and meeting those challenges head-on.

How This Book Is Organized

All *For Dummies* books are divided into parts and chapters. The goal is for you to easily move from one part or chapter to another without having to read a gazillion pages of information that aren't essential at the moment. Clever, right? The following sections describe each part.

Part I: Understanding PD

The chapters in this part explain what PD is and isn't. Chapter 1 gives an overview: statistics and background information plus the differences between primary PD and other conditions that can look like it. Chapter 2 gets into the potential causes—genetic and environmental—that researchers study to find new treatments and even a cure. You also find out who's at risk for getting PD. In Chapter 3 we take a closer look at the four major symptoms and signs that distinguish Parkinson's from related conditions. The chapter concludes with the stages of the disease and why these stages have no clear markers.

Part II: Making PD Part—But Not All—of Your Life

These chapters walk you through those initial steps following your suspicions of PD. We begin with guidance on getting an accurate diagnosis, finding a specialist, and understanding the tests and techniques that confirm your diagnosis. We explain how to connect with other health experts—therapists, counselors, and such—who will play a vital role in managing your PD. In addition, you need to focus on sharing the news with people around you. Chapter 7 gives you tips on how, when, and who to tell. The final chapter in this part addresses the special needs of people with young onset PD (before age 50).

Part III: Crafting a Treatment Plan Just for You

This is your guide to the current options for treating PD and managing symptoms over the long term. We look at prescription medicines, the possibility of surgery, and proven complementary or alternative therapies that are viable assets. The largest chapter is on diet and exercise, and that's intentional. We include a program of exercises specifically designed to enhance flexibility and build muscle strength. We also insist that you show this program to your physician and physical therapist before trying it on your own! Because PD is a neurological condition (affecting the brain), we include a separate chapter on depression and anxiety, which can be treatable symptoms of the condition itself. Wrapping up this part is a chapter on clinical trials. We discuss how to find such trials as well as the pros and cons of being a participant.

Part IV: Living Well with PD

Because living with PD for many years—even decades—is not only possible but also likely, this part discusses special areas of your life (people, work, and independence) that may need fine-tuning. We explain how people often react differently to a person who now has a chronic and progressive condition and how it's up to you to maintain normalcy with your family, friends, and co-workers. We also address PD and the workplace: the issues you face when you can work as well as the options you have when you can't work. Finally we cover ways to maintain independence and control over your life despite changes in your mobility and mental prowess.

Part V: Coping with Advanced PD

As with any progressive condition, you'll eventually delegate responsibilities and rely on other people to keep you mobile, mentally alert, and emotionally upbeat. This part of the book is as important for your primary care partner as it is for you, so both of you need to read it. We cover important decisions and planning processes that you should address early on, and we discuss the onset of later-stage symptoms that can be incapacitating. We also address the gradual shift of your partner's role from care partner to caregiver, based on ground rules the two of you make. Early discussions on housing, finances, and legal issues are also covered in this part.

Part VI: The Part of Tens

Every *For Dummies* book includes a section of lists, that is, key information that readers can use right away. In *Parkinson's Disease For Dummies,* those lists include ten ways to manage difficult feelings (anger, guilt, sadness, and such), ten ways you (the PWP) can care for your care partner, and—possibly the most important list—ten ways you and your care partner can become active in the fight for a cure.

Part VII: Appendixes

Appendix A contains a glossary of Parkinson's-related terms to use as reference. Appendix B summarizes the many PD resources we mention through-out this guide: organizations, care partner resources, support groups, and assistive devices for making life with PD easier.

Icons Used in This Book

To make this book easier to read and simpler to use, we include icons that help you find (and fathom) key information. Here's what they look like and highlight:

This icon flags essential information that cautions and protects you against potential pitfalls and problems. Do *not* skip over these paragraphs.

This icon signals essential information that's important enough to bear repeating. It's information you should keep in mind.

This icon identifies information that may save you time, offer a resource, or show you an easier way of doing some task or activity.

Where to Go from Here

Where you open this book—Chapter 1, Chapter 18, or somewhere in between—depends on where you are in your journey through Parkinson's. If you suspect PD is the cause behind some troubling symptoms, you may want to start with Chapter 4 for tips on the best way to get an accurate diagnosis. If you've already been diagnosed, then Part III, where we discuss treatment options, may be your first stop.

The point is that this is a *guide,* a roadmap to help you on the path to living with PD. We offer information and resources that you can trust—tools that help you adapt to life with PD without making it your whole life. In the long run, however, it's your resolve to face each day with renewed strength and energy that will see you through. And it's your example that will set the stage for those people who intend to partner with you in the fight.

Part I

Understanding PD

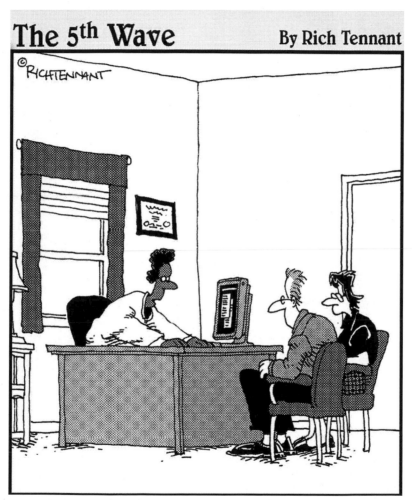

"As explained, Parkinson's disease is a depletion of dopamine in the brain. But before you fill up that space with a lot of negative thoughts, let's discuss your treatment options."

In this part...

You discover what Parkinson's disease is and how it differs from related forms of parkinsonism. We identify the current theories on causes for the onset of Parkinson's and the risk factors that may play a part for some people. Finally you get a good idea of what symptoms to watch for and what signs doctors look for to diagnose and stage this condition.

Chapter 1

Parkinson's Disease: The Big Picture

In This Chapter

• Setting the stage: What Parkinson's disease is—and isn't

• Making a plan to establish your care

• Maximizing your care options

• Living (and loving) your life

• Getting from here to there: Your present and future with PD

The National Center for Health Statistics (a division of the Centers for Disease Control) reports that approximately 1 percent of all Americans over the age of 65 receive a diagnosis of Parkinson's disease (PD). Sixty thousand new cases are diagnosed every year. But you didn't pick up this book because you're interested in mass numbers. You opened it because you're only interested in one number—yours or someone you love. You opened it because you've noticed some symptoms that made you think *Parkinson's,* or you just got a confirmed diagnosis and you're wondering what's next.

What's next is for you to go into action mode—understand the facts (rather than listen to the myths) about PD—what causes it, how it's treated, and, of huge importance to anyone diagnosed with PD, how to live with it. (Notice we said *live,* not just *exist.*) In this chapter, you find the big picture of the rest of the book and (more to the point) where to find the information that you need right now.

Defining Parkinson's—A Movement Disorder

Parkinson's disease is a disease in a group of conditions called *movement disorders*—disorders that result from a loss of the brain's control on voluntary movements. Dopamine (a neurotransmitter in the brain) relays signals from the substantia nigra to those brain regions (putamen, caudate, and globus pallidus—collectively named the *basal ganglia* —in the *striatum*) that control movement, balance, and coordination (see Figure 1-1). In the brain of people with Parkinson's (PWP), cells that produce this essential substance die earlier than normal.

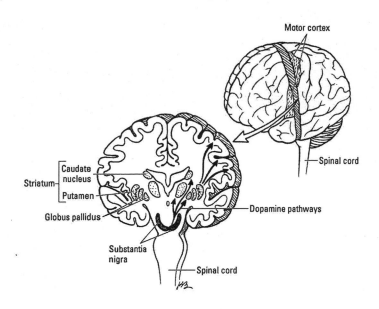

Figure 1-1: The dopamine pathway.

Although a whole group of conditions are known as *parkinsonism,* the one that most people know is called *idiopathic PD,* a Greek word that means arising spontaneously from an unknown cause. As the term suggests, the jury is still out as to the underlying cause (though theories do exist).

Go into a room filled with 50 people with Parkinson's (PWP) and ask how they first suspected they had PD. You're likely to hear 50 different stories. Take ten of those people who were diagnosed at approximately the same time and you're likely to see varying signs of PD progression—from almost no progression to more rapid onset of symptoms. Similarly, you're likely to experience a variety of attitudes and outlooks from the individuals dealing with their PD.

When you're diagnosed with PD, you set out on a unique journey—one where your outlook, lifestyle changes, and medical treatment can be key directional maneuvers along the way. In truth, this disease is one that you can live with, surrender to, or fight with everything you've got. The road veers and curves differently for each person. Some people may choose one path for managing symptoms, and some people choose another. Sometimes the disease itself sets the course. The bottom line? No clear roadmaps are available. But one fact is certain: Understanding the chronic and progressive nature of PD can take you a long way toward effectively managing your symptoms and living a full life.

Accepting the chronic progressive factors

Chronic and progressive can be scary words when you're talking about your health. But keep the words in perspective. Any number of chronic conditions occur with age—arthritis, high blood pressure, and cholesterol management to name three. So, take a realistic look at the terms, accept them for what they are (and aren't), and move on.

Chronic—it's part of you now

In medical terms, illnesses are either *acute* (develop quickly and usually go away with treatment or time) or *chronic* (develop over time, may be managed with treatment, but have no cure at this time). In short, a chronic illness like PD (or arthritis or high blood pressure) is now part of you—a fact that can help or hinder you in the fight.

If you refuse to accept that PD is a fact of life for you, then you're wasting precious time and energy in denial. But, if you accept that most people get challenges in life and PD is yours, then you're ahead of the game. Facing PD is no different than facing any situation that changed the way you thought your life would be.

Progressive—it will get more challenging

Progressive, advancing, worsening—more scary stuff. Here's some good news: For millions of PWP, the progression takes years, even decades. Many PWP live relatively normal life spans following their diagnosis. However, two factors are essential for successfully containing PD's progressive effects: your attitude and your willingness to attend to lifestyle and medical therapy.

Throughout this book we address both factors in multiple ways, but for now, remember:

- **Your attitude**—refusing to allow this diagnosis to color every part of your routine and life—is a huge factor in coping with the management of new symptoms through the years.

- **Your willingness to take lifestyle changes seriously** and get involved in the fight to find a cure can make all the difference between you managing the disease or the disease managing you.

To figure out how you're going to live with PD—if you have it—you first need to understand the basics: what it is (and is not), how you get it, what to look for, and how it progresses.

Distinguishing between Parkinson's disease and related conditions

Several neurological conditions may appear to be *idiopathic* (without known cause) PD at first, but they eventually trace back to known causes, progress differently, and respond differently to therapy. (Chapter 3 has more on this.) These other conditions include the following:

- **Essential tremor** (ET) is perhaps the most common type of tremor, affecting as many as five million Americans. ET differs from the tremor in idiopathic PD in several ways: ET occurs when the hand is active (as in eating, grasping, writing, and such). It may also occur in the face, voice, and arms. The renowned actress, Katherine Hepburn, had ET, not PD. Differentiating ET from PD is very important because each condition responds to completely different sets of medications.

- **Parkinson-plus syndromes** may initially have the same symptoms as PD. But these syndromes also cause early and severe problems with balance, blood pressure, vision, and cognition and usually have a much faster progression compared to PD.

- **Secondary parkinsonism** can result from head trauma or from damage to the brain due to multiple small strokes (*atherosclerotic* or *vascular parkinsonism*). Both forms can be ruled out through scans (CTs or MRIs) that produce images of the brain (see Chapter 4).

- **Pseudoparkinsonism** can appear to be PD when in fact the person has another condition (such as depression) that can mimic the inexpressive face of PWP.

- **Drug- or toxin-induced parkinsonism** can occur from taking antipsychotic medications (drug-induced) or from exposure to toxins such as carbon monoxide and manganese dust (toxin-induced). Drug-induced symptoms are usually (but not always) reversible; toxin-induced symptoms usually aren't.

The subtleties of diagnosing idiopathic PD may lead your family doctor to send you to a *neurologist,* a specialist in the treatment of neurological conditions. If that happens, don't panic. Getting the correct diagnosis, discussed in Chapter 4, is the first step toward figuring out what comes next for you.

Debunking some commonly held myths about PD

It's to your advantage to get a grasp on some of the more commonly held myths about PD—what it is and what it isn't.

- PD is not:

  - Contagious

  - Curable (at this writing, but research is hopefully getting closer!)

  - Normal for older people—or impossible for younger people

  - A reason to make immediate life-changing decisions (like assuming you won't be able to work or that you need to move)

  - Bound to get you if you live long enough

- PD is:

- Chronic (when you have it, you have it—like arthritis or diabetes)

- Slowly progressive (over time—often years) even with treatment

- Manageable (often for years) with proper treatment and key lifestyle changes

- Life-changing for you, your family, and friends (Whether that's good or bad is up to you and how you decide to face it.)

In many ways these debunkers are the key messages we want you to take away from this book. If you have PD, you have an enormous challenge before you, but tens of thousands of people successfully face it every day. You can get through this—and we're here to show you how.

Recognizing symptoms that raise questions

First things first: Do you have PD? Although researchers may not yet have a clear idea of the cause(s) for PD (see Chapter 3), they have established that idiopathic PD starts on only one side of the body and includes one or more of these four key symptoms:

- Tremor at rest (trembling in the hands, arms, feet, legs, or face when that body part isn't engaged in activity)

- Rigidity (stiffness in the limbs and trunk)

- Akinesia or bradykinesia (lack of movement or slowness of movement)

- Postural instability (impaired balance or coordination of movement)

Notice how the first letters of the symptoms spell out the handy acronym *TRAP* to help you remember (like you need to be reminded!). You'll have times when the symptoms of PD make you feel trapped inside your body. In this book, we work hard to show you a number of ways to fight back and maintain control of your life in spite of the *TRAP.*

Chapter 3 discusses symptoms (what you report to the doctor) and signs (what the doctor observes) in more detail.

Seeking the Care You Need

Perhaps more than any other chronic condition, managing PD is a team effort. You're going to be working with an entire front line of healthcare professionals (doctors, therapists, and the like) as well as non-professionals like your family and friends and other PWP that you'll meet along the way.

From medical professionals

At least two doctors are likely to be intricately involved: your primary care physician and a neurologist. In addition, you'll possibly connect with several other healthcare professionals along the way: your pharmacist; physical, occupational, and speech therapists; counselors and advisors to help manage any depression, anxiety, diet changes, and exercise regimens; advisors to help manage financial, legal, housing, and other major decisions that'll affect you and your family over the long term. Chapter 6 offers more information about this group.

From loved ones

You'll also have a personal care team: your spouse or significant other; your children (and possibly grandchildren); your close friends and (if you're diagnosed with young onset Parkinson's—YOPD) your parents and siblings. Benchwarmers who may surprise you with their willingness to help out include neighbors, co-workers, members of groups you belong to, and others. In Chapters 7 and 16 we talk more about how to break the news and get these folks involved. Chapter 8 covers questions and situations specific to YOPD.

As your PD progresses

One of the toughest truths you'll face as your PD progresses is that you have to rely on other people's help to some degree. Years may pass before this becomes a factor, but you and your loved ones need to plan for it. In Chapter 18 we discuss the symptoms that can crop up as your PD progresses. Every case of PD is different though; symptoms that occur in another person may never be a problem for you. Knowledge is good, but assuming that you'll have to endure every symptom in this book is just wrong on so many levels.

The more positive approach is to *prepare* without *projecting.* For example, will you have swallowing difficulties? Maybe, but you can have a speech therapist as a part your care team, as we talk about in Chapter 6. She's there on the bench, ready to get in the game if you need help. Will your spouse or significant other have to dress you, feed you, bathe you? Chances are good that he'll need to assist you in these basic daily activities in the advanced stages of your PD. We cover that step in Chapter 19.

Reaching decisions about advanced PD questions before they occur (such as identifying a caregiver and having a family meeting to plan an extended network of support) is just smart planning. (That's in Chapter 19 too).

Treating Parkinson's—Previewing Your Options

After you've educated yourself with facts (not myths or hearsay) and drafted your care team(s), it's time to get down to the serious business of treating your PD and managing symptoms as they appear. In this book we cover the options—in fact, a growing number of options—for treating and managing your PD symptoms. In addition to medications (Chapter 9) and—in some advanced cases—surgery (Chapter 10), you can find relief in complementary treatments (such as physical and occupation therapies) and alternative treatments (such as yoga or acupuncture). See Chapter 11 for more about all of these.

In the beginning your doctor may want you to post-pone a prescription-medication regimen in favor of trying some lifestyle changes—for example, diet and exercise (see Chapter 12) and counseling for your PD-related anxiety and depression (Chapter 13). With today's bright spotlight on research for a cure, you may even want to participate in one of the many clinical trials for new treatments (Chapter 14).

As new symptoms appear (usually years after your initial diagnosis), you'll want to check out Chapter 18 to understand the difference between symptoms that can be PD-related and symptoms that can be related to the aging process or another condition entirely(such as high blood pressure).

Starting the Course, Staying the Course

Not surprisingly, for many people and their families, the diagnosis of PD comes as a shock. *Progressive* and *incurable* are likely to be the words that register in these early hours. But as the news begins to sink in, you have choices to make. The following sections provide advice.

Dealing with the here and now

As Debi Brooks, President and CEO of the Michael J. Fox Foundation, notes in the foreword to this book, if you're going to truly have a life with PD, you need to do three things: develop an attitude of action, form a problem-solving mentality, and possess the ability to take a great deal of information coming at you from all directions and distill it into clear, logical next steps.

Here are some tips to get you on the road:

- Stay in the here and now—not the distant future. PD is a condition you can successfully manage, perhaps for many years, before you must rely on other people.

- Work with your healthcare team to focus on *your* PD and how you can most effectively manage those symptoms.

- Do *not* compare your situation, symptoms, or ability to manage to other PWP. This is not a contest and you are not those persons.

- Get organized. What are your questions? Write them down. Who are the best medical professionals to treat your PD? If finding that doctor means traveling to another community, at least consider it. This is your life, after all.

- Maintain some sense of control over your destiny by educating yourself. Use only reputable sources such as those we list throughout this guide and in Appendix B.

- Use the lingo. Everyone else will—your doctors, the people in your support group, the authors of the articles you read. We define terms as we go, but Appendix A is a glossary for your convenience.

- Be a team player by:

  • Taking the time to prepare for doctor appointments with questions and information about your current symptoms.

  • Taking charge of your own health by making changes to your diet and exercise routine as needed—and sticking with it.

• Understanding that, although you have every right to maintain independence and autonomy over your decisions, you also have a responsibility to care for the people who will care for and eventually speak for you.

• Encouraging innovation in your health team, your family and friends, and yourself. (For example, if you used to love playing jazz saxophone but your tremor makes that impossible, does that mean you have to give up loving jazz?)

• Celebrating even the smallest victory and allowing yourself a decent interval to mourn the greater losses.

• Remembering that your PD is not all about you. Other people are affected, some of them in major, life-changing ways.

• Advocating for new and more effective treatments and a cure. (You can't be more effective than when you're speaking out for those 60,000 PWP who are being diagnosed each year.)

• Learn as much as you can, lean on the support of other PWP who have been there (done that), laugh with other people and at yourself, love in return those people who offer love in their support and care, and LIVE with the single determination that you won't be reduced to a PD-only identification ("That's Jack Wilson—he's really an amazing person!").

Working, playing, and having a life

Okay, the medical experts are in place, you're on a regimen customized to manage your symptoms. What's next? How about getting a life—at least getting back to some semblance of the one you had before the diagnosis?

Part IV of this guide is all about living with PD: keeping up with the relationships that are so vital to you as an individual (Chapter 15), maintaining a job (even continuing to build a career if that's important for you; see Chapter 16), and getting out and about—you know, living (Chapter 17).

Making plans for your future

Any diagnosis of a chronic and progressive condition—no matter how slowly it progresses—is a wakeup call for attending to those financial and legal matters everyone needs to address. For you, that time is now. You and your family need to get together with an experienced team of financial and legal consultants and take steps to protect you and your loved ones in the event that you become incapacitated.

If at some point you can no longer speak for yourself or make the complex decisions in managing finances, your care partner must know your choices and have the power to act on your behalf. This advice is just common sense whether a person has PD or not. Chapter 20 offers guidelines and tips that can save you and your family a lot of stress and worry in the future on these matters.

If your current housing become an issue later on (for example bedrooms and the only bath are on the second floor), Chapter 21 takes a look at the growing range of options, including adapting your current residence so you can stay there.

In the course of our individual careers and our collaboration on this book, the three of us have seen case after case of people living full and satisfying lives in spite of PD. We understand that it isn't always easy, but we have seen the incredible results when PWP succeed in living beyond their disease.

Although no single resource can provide all the answers, we believe that in these pages you can find the information you need to make the best decisions for living your life with PD.

Chapter 2

Considering Possible Causes and Risk Factors

In This Chapter

• Understanding theories behind the possible causes of Parkinson's disease

• Determining risk factors

• Assessing your at-risk quotient

Although James Parkinson described the disease nearly two centuries ago and research has been ongoing ever since, the underlying cause—the factor that sets Parkinson's disease (PD) in motion—is still unknown. A number of theories are under discussion and research, any one of which may lead to the breakthrough in managing symptoms or even curing the disease. The medical community has also made progress in assessing risk factors—some more common than others. In this chapter we cover these potential causes and risk factors so you can better understand them as the hunt for a cure continues.

Considering Theories on Causes

The underlying event behind the onset of PD is a loss of neurons (nerve cells) in the *substantia nigra* region of the brain. These neurons normally produce *dopamine,* a neurotransmitter that helps the brain communicate with other parts of the body, telling them to perform common movements (such as walking, handling objects, and maintaining balance) almost automatically.

PD is a little like diabetes because in both diseases

- You lose a vital chemical (insulin in diabetes; dopamine in PD).

- The chemicals are essential to the body's ability to function properly.

- The chemicals can be replaced.

Of course, the diseases are more complex than that, but you get the idea. As we age, all of us lose dopamine-producing neurons, which results in the slower, more measured movements. But the decline of dopamine in people with Parkinson's (PWP) is not normal.

Why PD targets the substantia nigra at the stem of the brain remains a mystery. But the damage results in abnormal protein deposits that can disrupt the normal function of the cells in that area. These protein clumps are called *Lewy bodies,* named for Freiderich H. Lewy, the German physician who discovered and documented them in 1908. The presence of Lewy bodies within the substantia nigra is associated with a depletion of the brain's normal supply of dopamine. For this reason, their presence is one of the pathological hallmarks of PD (although Lewy bodies are present in other disorders).

In reality, Lewy bodies have been found in other parts of the brain affected by PD, which suggests that the problem may be more widespread. This more extensive pathology may explain the occurrence of non-motor and levodopa-unresponsive symptoms (see Chapter 9). Nevertheless, researchers still don't know whether Lewy bodies cause the damage to the nerve cells or are a by-product of damage caused by another factor.

Theories on causes abound—family history, environment, occupation, and so on. Today's researchers generally agree, however, that the onset of PD is a *multi-factorial* process; that is, several conditions are at play in the onset of PD rather than one specific and single cause. But the true causes behind the onset of PD in one person and not another—in one family member and not another—are unknown.

Much of the research today focuses on environmental and genetic factors that may contribute to the onset of PD. This section takes a look at those environmental conditions and then considers genetic issues and other factors that scientists have identified as potential causes.

Taking a close look at environmental factors

According to the National Institute of Environmental Health Sciences, PD is the second most prevalent neurodegenerative disorder behind Alzheimer's disease. Of the three primary risk factors for PD (age, genetics, and environmental exposures), a line of research that began in the 1980s shows an increasing association between environmental factors and PD. The following sections explore the variety of environmental exposures that may play a role in triggering PD.

Free radicals—the internal battle

Free radicals are unstable molecules that lack one electron. In their quest to replace that missing link, they rub against other molecules, seeking a connection that will stabilize them.

Even when the free radical doesn't make a connection, it keeps digging, damaging other molecules in the cell in a process known as *oxidation* or *oxidative stress.* Normally your body has enough antioxidants to stabilize the free radical and repair the damage, but if it doesn't, then those damaged cells die.

Key players in controlling oxidative stress are the *mitochondria* (the part of the cell outside the nucleus that converts nutrients into energy) because they're a potential source of free radicals. In addition, several of the toxins associated with PD seem to damage specifically the mitochondria. Researchers believe a connection may exist between oxidative stress and the death of cells in the substantia nigra, which causes PD symptoms. This theory is one of the main reasons that some doctors recommend a diet rich in antioxidants. (See Chapter 12 for more on diets for PWP.)

Location, location, location

For the overwhelming number of PD patients who get Parkinson's, certain environmental factors seem to put the person at higher risk for getting the disease. Consider that family members share not only a genetic history but also an environmental history—at least for a portion of their lives. They live in the same house, drink the same water, eat the same food from the same sources, have exposure to the same chemical compounds, and so on. Therefore, researchers are studying geographic environmental factors as a possible link to the onset of PD. These factors include living in a rural area and using well water for drinking, cooking, and such.

Exposure to toxins

Toxins that people inhale or ingest can damage the body in many ways, including cell function interference. Research shows that excessive exposure to specific environmental or industrial toxic chemicals such as pesticides and herbicides can increase the risk of developing PD. For example, the damage by the pesticide *rotenone* is directed at the *mitochondria* (the power plant of our brain cells) and can critically reduce the energy produced by the cell until the cell dies. (See the "Free radicals—the internal battle" sidebar for more on this topic.)

In some cases environmental toxicity and genetic factors may operate in tandem. Scientists have discovered that the gene CYP2D6, when functioning normally, produces an enzyme that breaks down the toxicity of pesticides.

But in some people the gene is less effective, leaving those people more sensitive to the toxicity of pesticides. More studies are needed to verify whether there may be a correlation between genetic predisposition to pesticide toxicity and PD.

Links to viral problems
Although PD is not contagious, a viral factor may be associated with its cause. This hypothesis is mainly based on the occurrence of *post-encephalitic parkinsonism* after the influenza pandemic of 1918. More Americans died from this flu in a single year than from the all the wars from World War I through the Vietnam War.

To complicate matters, many patients developed the so-called *sleeping sickness (encephalitis lethargica),* characterized by the progression from severe headache to drowsiness to possible coma and death. Patients who survived the encephalitis (brain infection) often developed symptoms of parkinsonism, including bradykinesia, rigidity, hypomimia, postural instability, and eye movement abnormalities *(oculogyric crises).* The memoir *Awakenings* by Oliver Sacks (Vintage) and the 1990 movie by the same title starring Robin Williams and Robert de Niro provide an insightful and accurate representation of this disease.

In reality, the relationship of a virus (such as influenza) and the brain degenerative lesions causing parkinsonism has not been proven. Furthermore, the pathology described in the brain of patients with post-encephalitic parkinsonism is very different from PD and actually bears more of a resemblance to Alzheimer's disease. So the possible viral link with parkinsonism remains elusive.

Although these environmental factors and cellular interactions appear to significantly contribute to the onset of PD, the Parkinson's Disease Foundation notes "no conclusive evidence that any single environmental factor, alone, can be considered a cause of the disease." (Go to the foundation's Web site at www.pdf.org/aboutPD/ and click on *Causes* for more information on this topic.)

Looking at possible genetic factors

Every human being plays host to a gazillion genes in their DNA molecules. Genes determine everything from the color of your eyes to the possibility of developing a certain disease or condition. Note the use of the word *possibility.* Because you carry genes in double copies, if one of your genes has the propensity for a condition, the other copy may offset that vulnerability.

According to the National Human Genome Research Institute, evidence now shows a genetic factor in the development of PD. People with a close relative (parent or sibling) who has PD are slightly more likely to contract Parkinson's than someone who has no family history of the disease. But, according to the Mayo Clinic, the link is a small one—less than 5 percent—and more common when the onset occurs before age 30, which is also very rare. (For more information on early onset PD, check out Chapter 8.)

So why waste time and money studying genes? Oddly enough, the very fact that PD is one of the most typical nongenetic diseases makes the genetic study of PD patients interesting. In other words, if PD is typically not inherited, then what else is going on?

In the last decade, scientists have identified multiple genes with definite links to the onset of PD in families where PD is present in multiple generations. An abnormality in one such gene, *Parkin,* may be a predictor of the onset of Parkinson's at a young age (before age 50). Because Parkinson's is present and progressing for several years before any symptoms become obvious, a gene predictor can mean earlier diagnosis and earlier intervention.

Another recent discovery shows that a *mutation* (change) in the protein-producing gene *alpha-synuclein* may change the gene's amino acid composition and thereby contribute to the development of *clumps* (separate cells bonding together) in dopamine neurons, eventually damaging or destroying the dopamine-producing neuron. Interestingly, alpha-synuclein is part of the Lewy bodies, the hallmark protein deposit in dopamine cells affected by Parkinson's disease. If researchers can find a way to break up those clumps and get rid of the excess proteins, then they may have found a way to slow or even stop the progression of PD. (See the section "Occupational causes" later in this chapter for more about clumping.)

Keep in mind that less than 5 percent of PWP appear to have inherited it; at this writing, any genetic factor seems limited to a relatively small number of families. However, the study of genes enhances the ability to understand which molecules a scientist may target for treatment. If you have a family history of PD or are interested in more information on genetic re-

search, visit www.ninds.nih.gov/disorders/parkinsons
_disease.

Checking out other possible causes

If it's not family history and it's not the environment, what caused your PD? Unfortunately, that's a difficult question to answer at this stage. And any time a chronic illness has no definitive cause, theories will fly. At the moment, PD has its fair share of such theories. The following sections describe instances where the jury is still out regarding a link with the onset of PD.

Latent effects of war
Links between PD and Agent Orange (an herbicide used during the Vietnam War) and chemical weapons during the Gulf War continue to be relevant questions for PD researchers. For example, in 2003 the Salk Institute identified a gene (called neuropathy target estrase or NTE). In studies with mice, scientists found that when NTE genes are exposed to organophosphate chemicals (such as those used in the Gulf War), the gene's normal activity was inhibited and even changed. While this discovery has certainly opened new doors (not to mention raised new questions), the evidence is far from conclusive. Remember that age is a consideration in the onset of PD and Vietnam vets are reaching the age that onset of PD is more common simply because of their generation. Whether exposure

to Agent Orange may also be a contributing factor is still not clear. The good news is that the Veterans Administration (VA) is conducting ongoing research. If you're a veteran of either war, you can find out more information by contacting the U.S. Department of Veterans Affairs online at www.va.gov.

Overmedication and drug use

Certain drugs taken to excess or over a long period of time may produce the symptoms of PD. Some of the conditions and their drugs include

- Schizophrenia, major depression, or agitation in older people: haloperidol (Haldol) and chloropromazine (Thorazine)

- Control of nausea: metoclopramide (Reglan) and prochlorperazine(Compazine)

Side effects of such medicines usually subside after the medicine is out of the body's system. **Note:** Symptoms brought on by drug use commonly occur on both sides of your body at the same time, unlike primary PD. The question remains whether a drug reaction of this nature is a predictor for PD.

Illicit drug use may also be a factor. In one case, a group of young people brewed up what they thought was a hallucinogenic drug called *meperidine* and mistakenly produced a heroin-like drug. When injected, this drug, which contained the toxin 1-methyl-4-phenyl-1,2,3,6-tetrahydropyridine (MPTP), headed straight for the substantia nigra, destroying dopamine cells in its path and leaving the youngsters with signs of advanced PD. The tragedy has led to more research on the possibility of a connection between illicit drug use and the onset of PD.

Occupational causes

Many people have theorized that Muhammad Ali's PD was brought on by his years in the boxing ring. "Too many times getting hit in the head," they assert. Indeed some studies suggest an association between head trauma and the development of PD. Possibly Ali's years in the ring brought the underlying presence of his PD to light.

Another class of work associated with onset of PD is the welding profession. At this writing, an absolute connection doesn't exist between prolonged exposure to metallic fumes or dust and the onset of PD-like symptoms. Nevertheless, researchers continue to explore the possibility of a link because studies show that exposure to heavy metals and pesticides—each already linked to a possible cause for onset of PD—can accelerate the clumping of certain protein cells called *alpha-synuclein.* (See the earlier section "Looking at possible genetic factors" for more on this gene.)

Sounds like sci-fi, but a word about neuroprotectors

The brain has two types of cells: *neurons* (nerve cells) and *glia* (cells that respond to injury and regulate the chemical composition surrounding them, among other tasks). Although glia cells are far more prevalent, the neuron cells do the heavy lifting when it comes to brain work. According to the National Institute of Neurological Disorders and Stroke, the three classes of neurons are:

• Sensory neurons to carry information from the senses (eyes, ears, and such) to the brain

• Motor neurons to carry messages from the central nervous system (comprised of the brain, spinal cord, and network of nerves running through the body) to the body's muscles and glands

• Interneurons that communicate only within their immediate location

Within each category, hundreds of neuron types operate with the very specific messaging abilities that make each person unique. But the neurons affected by PD control the body's ability to move. When those neurons die in large enough numbers, the brain's ability to signal the body to move is compromised.

Researchers are working hard to understand the death of these neurons and to develop treatments and therapies that can protect them. One potential value of stem cell research is that neural stem cells may reproduce the variety of neurons in the brain. Scientists could then figure out how to maneuver these new neurons to become

• A protector of healthy neurons (preventing or at least slowing further damage or loss)

• A replacement for damaged or dead neurons

In addition, ongoing research considers whether certain therapies—such as certain drugs, vitamin supplements, and rigorous exercise therapy—may act as a protector and slow the loss of these vital neurons. For more information on the role of neuro-

protection in the battle against PD, check out
Chapters 11 and 12.

Oddly enough, in more than one occupational study,
teachers and healthcare workers showed a higher incidence of PD—as much as two to three times higher
than other professions. Researchers are puzzled because the commonality in the two professions seems
to be exposure to infection, even though PD is clearly
not a contagious disease.

Weighing Your Risk Factors

Your suspicion that you have PD (or an actual diagnosis from your doctor) can raise all sorts of questions
starting with, "How did this happen to me?" It's perfectly normal to look back and consider the risk factors
that were present (although unknown at the time) as
you also look forward to protecting your children and
others around you from those same risks.

Start with what is known for sure:

- PD is not contagious—you can't get it from or give
  it to another person.

- Most cases (at least three-fourths) show up after
  age 60, and incidence increases every decade after
  that.

- Head trauma (a serious fall or accident involving injury to the head) can be a risk factor for PD.

- Men are more likely to get PD than women.

Your particular risk factors (or family members' risks if you suspect you have PD) are the life and lifestyle details that can increase the chances of developing PD. They may be *multi-factorial.* (You may be at risk from more than one source or situation).

Considering your age and gender

The one concrete risk factor for developing PD is age. Most people develop symptoms in middle age, but the risk for developing PD increases simply because dopamine production declines with age. The average age for onset is 60, and risk increases until around age 75. Some research has shown a significant decrease in the number of people who develop PD after age 75.

At least three studies have confirmed that men are more likely to develop PD than women—in some studies twice as likely. One theory suggests that the production of estrogen may protect women. At the 2006 meeting of the American Academy of Neurology, a research team from the Mayo Clinic presented evidence that points to a possible link between risk for contracting PD and three genes that control the production of estrogen. Simply put, if the presence of estrogen reduces the risk, a decrease in estrogen increases a woman's risk factor for getting PD. However, more studies are needed to confirm a protective role for estrogen in PD.

Taking a look at ethnicity

Studies have shown that non-white populations, such as African Americans and Asian Americans, have a lower risk of developing primary Parkinson's disease but may be more vulnerable to other forms of parkinsonism such as essential tremor and multiple system atrophy (see Chapter 1). However, whether this difference is tied to an economic and class-based imbalance in the delivery of medical care—especially specialized medical care, like seeing a neurologist—has not been fully considered.

Regarding other risk possibilities

Although they aren't definitive causes, some factors we discuss in this chapter may contribute to your risk for developing PD. In a world where pesticides and herbicides have so many uses, it's hard to avoid exposure to chemicals that put you at risk for all sorts of health problems including PD. Similarly, in an eat-on-the-run fast-food society, people may be denying their body's needs for key vitamins and nutrients. And what about the dangers of such evils as smoking and caffeine? Can these all be factors that put people at greater risk for getting PD?

Overexposure to herbicides and pesticides
Your everyday exposure to chemical toxins can range from the chemicals to control weeds on your lawn to the unseen sprays that coat and polish fresh produce from overseas. Because prolonged or consistent exposure to such toxins is a possible cause of PD (check out "Taking a close look at environmental factors" early in this chapter for more on toxins), take the following precautions:

- Wash all fresh produce thoroughly—even those items like melons or citrus where you normally discard the skin.

- Limit your exposure to the use of toxins such as pesticides and insecticides.

- Use all chemical materials in open areas and wear a protective mask.

If your job requires you to work with chemical compounds such as those in industrial pesticides and herbicides, talk to your employer about precautions to protect you and other employees from exposure and contamination.

Factoring in your weight

Face it: Being overweight sets you up for all kinds of health risks. A 2002 study showed that carrying excess weight during your middle and later years can put you at greater risk for PD. A report in the May, 2003 issue of *Psychology Today* magazine shows an increased rate of PD linked to dietary fat and sugar intake. Although the association between weight gain and PD hasn't been proven, the benefits of a diet rich in antioxidants and a regular program of exercise can't hurt. (In some cases, these benefits have prolonged the time before PD symptoms needed to be treated with medication (see Chapter 12).

Reduced levels of B6, B12, and folate

B6, B12, and folate are essential nutrients for maintaining many of the body's functions. Researchers are beginning to explore whether reduced levels of these nutrients may be a factor in PD. Although studies are in preliminary stages to verify any role the nutrients may play in the management of PD, consider asking your doctor about increasing or supplementing your intake of nutrients.

Regardless of the research and the nutrients' potential for managing your PD, people over age 50 are at increased risk for deficiencies of these three essential nutrients. A diet rich in these nutrients and a supplement (if your doctor advises) may be helpful. However, these need to be carefully monitored by your doctor. Too much B6, for example, can cause additional neuropathic problems such as a profound inability to feel your legs.

Check with your doctor before taking any vitamin or herbal supplement. Claims for these products often lack solid research. The overuse of such products may do more harm than good.

Smoking and caffeine

Get this: As many as 50 published studies over two decades have shown that smoking cigarettes reduces the risk of Parkinson's in people who have smoked steadily most of their adult lives. Caffeine also appears to offer some protection.

But these factors are not a guarantee (as Michael J. Fox noted in an NBC *Dateline* interview in 2006). And the negative effects of these factors (such as lung cancer from smoking) that can greatly shorten your stay on this planet are way too grim to think a two-pack-a-day habit may be worth the risk.

Changing Don't Know to Know

The more researchers tackle the problems of PD, the more complex the challenges become. This section takes a quick look at the unknowns of PD and offers ways that PWP and the general public can help PD research move forward.

The need-to-know info

Questions for PD researchers abound, but one of the greatest challenges is simply getting a good handle on the accurate numbers and extent of PD. For example

- Scientists really don't know how common Parkinson's is.

- They don't know whether the numbers are changing over time or simply reflecting longevity and an aging population.

- They don't know whether geographic cluster patterns exist (places in the United States where PD is unusually prevalent or absent).

The Muhammad Ali Foundation has established a voluntary registry where patients may record their PD diagnosis and information. (Register at

> www.alicenter.org.) However, because this informa-
> tion is random and voluntary, it has limited practi-
> cality.
>
>
> TIP

At this writing, PD has no national registry where doctors can report the diagnosis of PD in the United States. (California is the only state where doctors must report cases of Parkinson's.) A mandatory national registry for the diagnosis of PD would be an enormous step forward (a global registry would be even better!) and one of the best ways to help researchers gather the knowledge and data they need. This registry may seem an invasion of your privacy, but information that allows researchers to track patterns is the best way to gain vital knowledge that leads to new treatments and a cure.

The attitude that busts research barriers

At the 2006 World Parkinson's Congress in Washington, D.C., Joan Samuelson (founder of the Parkinson's Action Network) said that when first diagnosed, she believed her job was to be a *patient patient.* That attitude quickly changed as Joan understood more about the known and unknowns of PD. Today her motto is that patients need to be *in the room*—the PD patient community needs to take a vocal and proactive role in helping research move forward.

You may not be ready to take on this larger fight, but keep it in the back of your mind as you use this book. **Note:** In many ways you've taken a key first step—you're educating yourself about Parkinson's and what a diagnosis may mean for you and your loved ones. But getting involved with the greater Parkinson's community at a local, state, and national level is one of the most empowering steps you can take to live a full and productive life in spite of PD. (And when you are ready to get more involved, see Chapter 14 for more information on clinical trials and Chapter 24 for ideas on advocacy roles.)

Chapter 3

Sizing Up Symptoms, Signs, and Stages

In This Chapter

- Getting the terms straight

- Taking stock of your symptoms

- Prioritizing: Primary and secondary signs

- Categorizing the progression of PD

- Keeping the care partner in the loop

Whenever you have a concern about your health, you've usually taken note of certain troubling (and unexplained) symptoms. Perhaps you seem more clumsy than usual or your joints seem unusually stiff and rigid. If these symptoms are troubling enough, you're likely to make an appointment with your primary care physician (PCP) to have them checked out. After you describe your symptoms, your doctor conducts a clinical exam looking for signs that may explain your symptoms.

In this chapter, we describe the *symptoms* that can signal Parkinson's disease (PD) as well as the *signs* your doctor looks or to reach a diagnosis. Although many chronic, progressive conditions move through defined stages, this chapter stresses how progression in PD is unique for each patient.

Familiarizing Yourself with the Lingo

In the medical world, a *symptom* is

- What you feel or perceive before you see the doctor.

- The reason you ultimately decide to make an appointment.

- The details (vague or specific) you give when the doctor or nurse asks why you've come in.

For example, you may say that you're more tired than usual or moving more slowly because you lack energy. Or perhaps you're depressed or experiencing dizziness or shaking.

In contrast, medical *signs* are what your doctor observes during the examination. The best doctors use their senses in addition to the data from the usual medical imaging techniques and screening tools (see Chapter 4 for more about these instruments). For example, a doctor's touch may sense tightened muscles, or his eyes may observe a fine tremor when your hand's at rest, or he may note a compromised balance or slight shuffle when you walk. His ears may detect softer speech, a searching for words, or unusual sounds in your lungs or intestines.

Simply put, symptoms make up your subjective report of your experiences, and signs contribute to your doctor's objective basis for a diagnosis.

Disease *staging* divides a chronic and progressive illness into levels that usually correspond to the advancement of symptoms and disease. Generally, stages have the following labels:

- *Early stage:* The disease is manageable with little outside assistance.

- *Moderate stage:* The patient needs more assistance and lifestyle changes.

- *Advanced stage:* The disease has advanced to the point that can be difficult to manage; the patient may face the end of life.

The following sections take a closer look at symptoms (what you tell your doctor), signs (what your doctor observes and discovers via tests and examination), and staging (where you are in the progression if you do have PD).

Symptoms—What You Look for

Let's cut to the chase. You suspect that you or someone you love may have PD or you wouldn't be flipping through this book and you definitely wouldn't have turned to this chapter. Ask yourself what's behind those suspicions.

- **A slight shakiness in the hands?** Does it occur in only one hand? If the shaking occurs while the hand is at rest, does it stop when that hand picks up a cup of coffee, a pen, or a tennis racket? If the shakiness is in both hands and doesn't stop when the person grasps something, then PD probably isn't the cause (but get it checked out anyway).

- **A general slowing down of movement?** Does it take longer to walk from one place to another or to get in and out of the car? Has there been an increase in stumbling, clumsiness, or loss of balance? Do you (or does the person) feel tired, stiff, or just not *yourself*?

- **A significant change in energy level or out-look?** Everyone experiences days when they're tired or weaker than usual. And everyone has the blues from time to time. But if you've been feeling unusually weak, fatigued, depressed, or anxious for longer than two weeks, those symptoms need attention—even when you have a plausible cause (such as an unusually busy week at work or the death of a loved one).

- **Gastrointestinal problems (like constipation) or psychological problems (like increased nervousness or anxiety)?** In some cases, patients show none of the usual symptoms, so don't stop with the more traditional PD symptoms.

These are the symptoms—the feelings, aches, and pains that have made you think something's not right. It may be PD or it may not. Either way, you owe it to yourself to get your doctor's assessment.

Signs—What Your Doctor Looks for

When you see your doctor, she'll listen as you describe your symptoms and then conduct an examination to determine what those symptoms indicate. As you talk about your symptoms, your doctor begins a *differential diagnosis* if your symptoms indicate several possibilities. For example, if your symptoms are in keeping with PD, your doctor also looks for signs that indicate PD. But any doctor worth her salt doesn't offer a firm diagnosis before she's seen the results of several tests and a specialist has confirmed her suspicions.

In addition to four primary signs of PD (which may or may not be evident when you first go to the doctor), your doctor considers several secondary signs and symptoms. And because PD is a neurological condition, it doesn't just affect your physical movement; it can also trigger non-motor or cognitive signs and symptoms. We discuss all of these signs and symptoms in the following sections.

Four primary signs

Although the actual causes and risk factors for getting PD are still mysterious (see Chapter 2 for more on these factors), the primary signs that signal the presence of PD are very clear. You may have noticed one or more of these signs but then dismissed it as something slight, easily explained, or due to an entirely different condition.

Several resources use the acronym *TRAP* to illustrate the four primary signs of PD. And, because PD seems to trap your body with your brain's compromised ability to communicate, the acronym makes the top four symptoms easy to remember.

T=Tremor at rest (uncontrolled shaking)

PD was originally called *shaking palsy* because the *resting tremor* (it goes away as soon as the hand is engaged) rarely occurs in other illnesses. Characteristically, the resting tremor begins in one hand and moves to the other hand years later in the disease. The tremor may extend to the leg or foot on the same side and sometimes to the lips and jaw—or you may have no tremor at all. Tremor in the head and neck, however, is less common in primary Parkinson's disease.

Variations of the resting tremor include:

* Postural tremor (obvious when arms are extended to hold a position or posture)

* Action tremor (present when certain tasks, such as holding, are performed)

* Internal tremor (the patient feels the tremor but can't show it, almost as if it's coming from inside)

While tremor is the most obvious symptom of PD, it doesn't have to be present for diagnosis.

R=Rigidity (stiff muscles)

Rigidity is probably the most ignored and easy-to-explain-as- something-else sign. In plain English, *rigidity* means *stiffness.* (Who doesn't experience stiffness in joints and limbs that makes movement more difficult as they age?) If your doctor observes rigidity (without other signs of PD), he may first suspect arthritis and prescribe an anti-inflammatory medication. But, if medicine doesn't relieve the stiffness, you need to let your doctor know.

A=Akinesia (absence or slowness of movement)

Especially early on, people with PD (PWP) may experience slight *bradykinesia* (unusually slow movement). Much later in the progression, that slowed movement may become *akinesia* (no movement).

Get to know these terms because, if indeed you or a loved one has PD, you'll hear these words again and again. *Kinesia* means *movement* in the sense of knowing what you want your body to do. So *akinesia* and *bradykinesia* indicate problems initiating or continuing an action. For example, to walk across the room, you stand up and your brain tells your foot to step out—but with bradykinesia, your body doesn't move right away.

The problem can extend well beyond simply walking from here to there. Bradykinesia can also affect

- Facial expression because it slows blinking eye movement and the ability to smile. Read more about this *facial mask* in the next section, "Secondary signs and symptoms."

- Fine motor movements, such as the ability to manage buttons or cut food because the fingers lack the necessary speed and coordination to perform these detailed actions. In addition, fingers may curl or stiffen because of rigidity.

- The ability to easily turn over in bed because of lack of coordination between the various parts of the body that need to move in sequence; again muscle stiffness and rigidity may further complicate this normally routine task. (See discussion of secondary signs and symptoms later in this chapter.)

P=Postural instability (impaired balance)
In a healthy person, the natural movement is to alternately swing the arms and step forward with assurance. For PWP, however, the swing slowly decreases; in time the person moves with small, uncertain, shuffling steps. (PWP may adapt by propelling themselves forward with several quick, short steps.) Other PWP experience episodes of *freezing* (their feet feel glued to the floor).

Problems with balance (resulting in falls that can cause major injuries, hospitalization, and escalation of symptoms) are usually not a factor until later stages in PD. In time, PWP may lose the ability to gauge the necessary action to regain balance and prevent a fall. They may grasp at doorways or other stationary objects in an effort to prevent the loss of balance. Unfortunately, these maneuvers can make PWP appear to be under the influence of alcohol or other substances.

Secondary signs and symptoms

Many of the following indicators—although not essential to a PD diagnosis—are observable early on and can contribute to the diagnosis of PD. During your appointment, tell your physician anything that is troublesome regarding these secondary symptoms. They're part of your symptomatic history that helps your doctors see the total picture of your condition.

Facial mask

The mask (lack of facial expression) is a common sign of PD, and it can lead people to assume that you're not listening or not understanding the conversation. The difference may simply be a change in your facial expression due to decreased animation or emotion. Maybe someone has said, "You don't smile as often," and you're thinking, "I'm smiling just as often as before!" Likewise, people may accuse you of staring, but the real problem is that the number of eye-blinks has decreased.

Slowed or slurred speech

You (or other folks) may notice that your voice is softer or fades away after a strong start. Your doctor may further note that your voice lacks normal variations of tone and emotion or that you sound hoarse but report nothing to explain that hoarseness. In some cases you may have trouble saying a word clearly; you slur it instead of enunciating.

As PD advances, other speech issues (such as stuttering or speaking very rapidly) can appear;

swallowing difficulties may develop later in the disease. (See Chapter 18 for more info about advanced symptoms of PD.)

Small, cramped handwriting

Handwriting that once was free-flowing and smooth may appear increasingly cramped and jerky. This *micrographia* typically appears as letters that become progressively smaller (for example: *Parkinson*) and closer together.

Constipation and urinary incontinence

Most people (even some doctors) associate constipation with aging. But PD can also slow the bowels (as it does the rest of the body), so mention any unusual changes in bowel habits or routine to your doctor.

By the same token, *urinary frequency* (having to urinate often) and *urinary urgency* (NOW!) are common sideshows in the aging process. Although these problems may be signs of a totally unrelated condition, they are not uncommon in PD. Definitely bring these symptoms to your doctor's attention.

Increased sweating or oily skin

A sensitivity to heat and cold and excessively oily (or dry) skin are other signs that may indicate PD.

Non-motor signs and symptoms

Although the *TRAP* signs (check out the earlier section, "Four primary signs") are often enough evidence to raise the possibility of PD, non-motor factors may be present before those primary signs appear. Your doctor may ask questions to discover underlying symptoms that you've been ignoring or simply discounting.

It is vital that you keep an open mind and answer your doctor's questions as honestly and fully as possible. Any one of the following symptoms or a combination of them may indicate a condition other than PD. Don't jump to conclusions or try to self-diagnose. Trust your doctor on this!

Anxiety or depression

Anxiety and depression are such an integral part of PD that they get their own chapter (Chapter 13) in this book. For now, remember that these feelings may be some of the earliest symptoms of PD. Anxiety episodes can range from a mild, underlying feeling of uneasiness to a full-blown panic attack. Depression may disguise itself as a general lack of interest in normal activities, or it may be severe enough for you or your family to consider counseling or medication.

Executive dysfunction and cognitive abnormalities
Do you have trouble balancing your checkbook, following directions, or making decisions? In medical terms, these symptoms are examples of *executive dysfunction.* Another term, *cue-dependent function,* is also part of the non-motor symptom package, and it means you need a reminder of some sort. For example, you may need an alarm that tells you to take your medicine or attend a meeting. Or you have labels on cabinets and drawers to remind you of their contents. Of course, many people use these re-minders, especially when their lives are jammed with multiple responsibilities and a calendar brimming with appointments and commitments. But if you notice an escalation in the need for such reminders, mention it to your doctor.

In addition as many as half of all PWP experience problems with memory, thought processing, and word finding. These symptoms are usually more pronounced in later stages (see Chapter 18).

Dizziness or lightheadedness
In some cases dizziness or lightheadedness is due to a drop in blood pressure when you stand up, especially in warm weather or over-heated rooms. Although dizziness can be a factor in a number of conditions,

don't ignore mentioning it to your doctor if it's one of your symptoms.

Sleep disturbances

PWP usually have no trouble getting to sleep. The more common problems are staying asleep, napping throughout the day, and moving restlessly when asleep. In some cases, the PWP has intense dreams that add to the restlessness and disturbance of normal sleep.

Sexual dysfunction

As with many medical conditions, PD can adversely affect sexual desire and performance. The underlying causes may or may not be related to PD; however, if the problem is part of your PD, it may be relieved with proper medication and treatment.

Visual hallucinations

Visual hallucinations (seeing people or objects that really aren't present) can be a side effect of many medications. In the case of antiparkinsonian meds, hallucinations are usually benign. **Note:** If a patient reports hallucinations before the PD diagnosis and before she begins taking PD meds, the doctor will look for other medications or causes that may be at the root of the problem.

Stages—Understanding the Unique Path PD Can Take

The key to living with any chronic, progressive illness is taking responsibility to maintain your life beyond that condition. We discuss this in much greater depth throughout the book. For now, the significant question is: If this is PD and it does progress, then how fast and to what extent?

Some *chronic* (long-lasting) and *progressive* (advancing or worsening) diseases have clear-cut divisions between *stages* (obvious and even predictable changes in the patient's condition). However, PD isn't one of those—it affects each patient differently. In rare cases, PD can progress rapidly; the person quickly becomes dependent on others for assistance with basic daily activities. However, for most PWP the progression takes years. With proper treatment and management of new symptoms, PWP can live independently for quite some time before they need close care.

Don't let yourself or others try to project the future. *Prepare*—plan for what may happen—yes. *Project* —assume it will happen on a certain timetable—no. Projecting only adds to your anxiety and may actually prevent you from taking some measures that prolong the time between stages.

In spite of PD's lack of clearly defined and timed steps, your doctor may describe your condition in terms of stages. This breakdown is common practice in the medical profession because it permits doctors to use a common and accepted language when making notes about your condition. If you need to change doctors midstream, the new physician's ability to understand the previous doctor's notes can save you valuable time and enhance the new doctor's ability to address your needs.

Although your PD takes a path unique to you and in response to your lifestyle and medical choices, the disease does have some broad outlines of progression. For a fuller discussion of PD rating scales that determine its various stages, turn to Chapter 4.

Early stage PD: When life can be fairly normal

You may have experienced (and ignored) certain warning signals from PD for several years before you went to your doctor. Maybe you were constantly tired or had a vague, don't-feel-good sensation. As your general movement slowed, maybe you dismissed it as *getting older* or *lack of energy today.*

Then you began to notice some troubling (not to mention, annoying!) symptoms: stiffness that was different from the not-as-young-as- I-used-to-be version, shakiness, dizziness, or mood changes. You know the list.

If you have tremor, you may have barely noticed it at first, or maybe you dismissed it as a spasm. It may have appeared in one finger, so you noticed it only when you were performing a certain task, like tying your shoe or buttoning a jacket.

In *early* stage PD, the following conditions may occur:

• Symptoms are mild and often easily explained.

66

- Symptoms are annoying when they occur, but they don't significantly interfere with normal activity.

- Symptoms occur on only one side of the body.

- Tremor is present in one limb—usually the hand—and is most noticeable when the hand is at rest.

- Other people may comment on changes related to appearance, posture, energy, and facial expression.

In the early stages of PD, you can manage for some time with no pharmacological intervention. In other words, you don't need pills to control the symptoms.

Moderate stage PD: When you need to accept help

The defining signal of progression in PD is symptoms on both sides of the body. However, even at this stage, the diagnosis of PD has been missed in some cases simply because the symptoms (rigidity, gait change, tremor) were taken as normal signs of aging.

Other factors that may signal the *moderate* stage include the following:

- Your posture becomes stooped; your head is more often bent forward with your chin toward the chest.

- Movement of all body parts is significantly slower. When you walk, you often experience *freezing* (your feet feel glued to the floor); your hand tremor may now affect your entire arm, making activities such as shaving or brushing your teeth more difficult.

- Cognitive and executive function (see "Non-motor signs and symptoms" earlier in this chapter) is more impaired. Short-term memory, putting thoughts into words, balancing a checkbook, and making decisions are all more challenging.

- *Late-moderate* denotes increasing need for anti-dopaminergic medications. Problems with balance and risks of falls (which may result in injuries that require hospitalization) can actually speed the onset of late stage PD. (See Chapter 17.)

- PWP must rely on medicines as well as assistance from other people to pursue many of the activities they took for granted before PD. Examples of these activities are driving, getting in and out of a chair or bed, and going to the bathroom.

As symptoms progress, the challenging task for you and your doctors will be to manage your symptoms (see Chapter 9).

After you begin taking them, antiparkinsonian medicines can be amazingly effective. But they also have some serious and unsettling side effects. (For more about PD meds and their side effects, check out the discussion in Chapter 9.) Balancing the dosages and timing is a constant challenge that becomes more difficult as you move from the moderate to the late stage. The good news is that new medicines become available every year, medicines that—ideally—can be more effective without the frustrating side effects.

Late stage PD: When planning keeps you in control

When a PWP reaches the point of serious disability (that is, unable to lead a normal, independent life without major assistance), the medical community describes the stage as *late* or *advanced.* At this stage even the medications that were working so well in the earlier stages start creating problems and complications, and unless the PWP is a candidate for deep brain stimulation surgery (see Chapter 10), he may face unprecedented challenges. This is the stage (for most patients, it's years after the initial diagnosis) when all your planning and preparing (that we preach about throughout this book) pays off for you and your family. In spite of advancing frailty, you are still in control. You have made the decisions necessary to see you through this time, and your family understands and accepts your wishes. You can probably guess the signs:

- Walking is possible only with a walker and for short distances, if at all.

- The entire body is stiff and rigid; balance is significantly compromised.

- The PWP can no longer manage without considerable assistance.

- Cognitive impairments worsen; physical limitations increase.

- The benefits of medication wear off earlier between each dose.

- The PWP is usually confined to bed and requires round-the-clock care (most advanced stage).

The length of each stage is unique to each PWP. With lifestyle and medical therapies and even with certain interventions along the way, PWP can maintain the early-stage status quo for several years.

A Few Words for You and Your Care Partner

If you're living with someone that you suspect has PD, encourage that person to seek a definitive diagnosis. The symptoms may or may not be PD. Many symptoms associated with PD are also factors in illnesses and conditions that are treatable and curable. Neither you nor the other person should jump to conclusions, but you shouldn't ignore the warning signs either.

If the diagnosis is PD, then your first job is to understand that this person you love can continue to live an independent and self-reliant life for some time, even many years.

If you're the person's care partner:

- Don't assume you need to be Super-Caregiver. Resist the urge to go into full-on nurturing mode; encourage independence and self-reliance.

- Understand that adding PD to your already busy life can lead to problems if you aren't proactive and don't take the necessary steps to integrate your new role into the rest of your life.

- Be aware that a decline in the PWP's self-reliance and confidence may be a sign of depression—a common symptom of PD.

If you're the PWP:

- Maintain your independence and refuse to permit PD to rob you of the normal roles you've always played in all your relationships.

- Understand that depression is perfectly normal when you first hear that you have PD; however it is not normal for such depression to be pro-longed to the point that it actually escalates the progression of your PD and your need for hands-on care.

For each of you, the second task is to realize (and accept) that all the medicines and physician advice in the world can't be effective unless the PWP follows treatment recommendations, including changes in lifestyle. Self-management (the ability to take responsibility through changes in attitude and behavior) is the key to living with chronic illness of any type—and vital for living with PD. If you're the partner, consider what changes you can make in your own routines and habits that support and encourage the PWP to fight this disease.

The following tips may help both of you cope in these early stages:

- Find out everything you can—from reliable and respected sources—about PD. (See Appendix B for many of the best resources.)

- Ask questions. Chapters 4 and 5 deal specifically with the diagnosis and the steps immediately following it.

- Take an active role in partnering with the PWP and medical professionals to consider treatment options and manage symptoms (See Chapter 6 for teaming up with the pros and Chapters 9, 10, and 11 for more about treatment options.)

- Maintain emotional balance as you each cope with your fears and anxieties about the meaning of this diagnosis for you and other people close to the PWP. (Chapter 7 offers ideas on dealing with other people. Chapters 15 and 19 address relationship questions you may be asking.)

- Remind each other of times when the PWP faced a difficult situation and didn't just cope, but triumphed in handling it.

- Whether you're the PWP or the care partner, don't wait to get help for obvious anxiety and depression. (Chapter 13 covers this piece of PD in more detail.)

If the diagnosis is PD, don't panic. You and the PWP are now members of a unique, extraordinarily proactive, well-organized community. If you open yourself to that community, you'll be richer for the friends you make, the information you exchange, and the comfort you share.

Part II

Making PD Part—But Not All—of Your Life

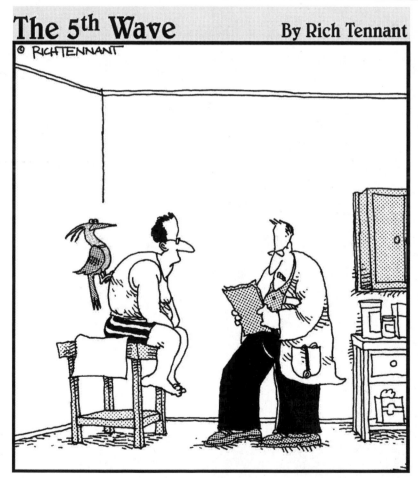

"Parkinson's disease? Well, maybe. But, like that pain in your shoulder, it could be a lot of things."

In this part...

We explore the intricacies of making an accurate diagnosis and why you should see a specialist—a neurologist—to develop a plan for treating your PD and managing your symptoms. You get the basics on how to assemble the healthcare support team you're going to need and the best way (and time) to let other people know of your diagnosis. This part includes a special chapter filled with information for people under age 50 who have young onset Parkinson's disease (YOPD).

Chapter 4

Getting an Accurate Diagnosis

In This Chapter

• Prepping for your primary care doctor

• Partnering with a neurologist

• Understanding the diagnosis process

• Looking for a second opinion

Okay, perhaps you've checked out Chapters 2 and 3 to see the causes and risk factors of Parkinson's disease (PD) as well as its signs and symptoms. And maybe the more you read, the more you worried that you (or someone you care for) may actually have it. Before you freak out, get to a doctor and find out for sure. Your imagination about PD and its consequences is far worse than living with it. In reality, many people with PD live relatively normal and fully active lives for many years after diagnosis. It's your call, but you can set this book aside right now and go bury your head in the sand, or you can take a measured, proactive approach to checking out those symptoms.

Ah, you're still here—great! (Okay, so the book's a little sandy. No problem.) The first step is to get an accurate diagnosis of your symptoms, starting with an accurate list of your current symptoms and medical history. Follow that with a visit to your primary care physician (PCP), who may recommend that you see a specialist. No doubt, you'll be prodded and tested, but you'll finally have a diagnosis. Last step? You want to get that diagnosis confirmed. Ready? Here we go.

Bringing Up the Subject with Your Doctor

This isn't going to be the usual appointment with your doctor. You're not going for an annual checkup or some routine test. You're making this appointment because you have symptoms that you can't explain and that don't seem to be going away. And you're making this appointment because you're concerned something is seriously wrong. An appointment for these reasons needs careful planning all along the way, from scheduling the appointment to gathering information to preparing questions you want to ask. All of this needs to happen *before* the appointment.

Scheduling an appointment

When you call your doctor's office to schedule the appointment, ask to speak to the doctor's nurse or assistant. Tell that person why you're scheduling the appointment. (Yes, go ahead and say it, "I'm concerned that I may have Parkinson's disease.") Then add that you want an appointment when the doctor will have more time—especially if your suspicions are correct. Also ask the nurse what information you should bring with you. When you do make the appointment (usually through the office manager or receptionist), only you can weigh the possible wait (perhaps several weeks until the doctor has this extra time) against the earliest available appointment. **Note:** If you choose the latter, consider booking that later appointment as well in case you want to follow up in more detail with the doctor. In either case, ask to be on the call list. In the event of a cancellation, you can then get to see the doctor sooner.

Preparing for your initial exam

Before seeing your PCP, plan to take the following steps to make that first meeting as productive as possible.

Gathering your medical records
First, be sure that your PCP has copies of all medical records. For example, if you've been seeing a cardiol-

ogist, your PCP needs copies of any lab work or stress test results as well as that doctor's notes on observations and treatment.

As soon as you schedule the appointment with your PCP, ask the office staff of any specialist you're seeing to fax copies of recent lab results to your PCP's office. Preparing and transferring such information can take time. So, if time is short, call the clinic where the tests were done or the doctor who ordered the tests and ask for a copy of the results. Then you can pick up these reports and take them with you to your appointment.

Prioritizing your symptoms

Next, make a list of your symptoms and prioritize them. For example, maybe the following is your list of symptoms:

- Anxious and not my usual upbeat self

- Shaky—especially in my right hand

- Unusually fatigued—no get-up-and-go

- Not sleeping well

If you suspect PD because you've noticed a slight tremor, you may want to move the second bullet (shaky) to the top of your list.

Keep in mind that the doctor's staff may interview you first. When the nurse asks you why you came in, the first words out of your mouth get her attention. So, if you say, "I haven't been sleeping that well," rather than "Over the last few weeks I've noticed a slight shakiness in my right hand," the nurse writes that your primary issue is *sleep disturbance.* And that statement can take matters in a whole different direction, wasting precious time.

Your doctor refers to the first symptom as your *chief complaint.* When she follows up on your answer with some form of "What makes you suspect Parkinson's?" then you can offer the rest of the symptoms on your list.

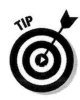

For heaven's sake, if you suspect PD, don't be afraid to introduce it into the conversation right away. Life—and doctor's appointments—are too short to beat around the bush!

Compiling your medical history

Writing down your personal medical history helps you prepare for the many questions along the way to your diagnosis. Preparing your history in advance also gives you time to think carefully about the specifics instead of trying to remember details on the spot.

If you've seen a doctor recently, you know that the questions are usually the same—no matter how many times you give the information. First, one or two members of the staff gather your information, and then the nurse or physician assistant (PA) may ask the same questions. But, with a trusty print-out of your history, you can provide a clean copy for their file and still have a copy in-hand (you made two copies, right?) to prompt you on dates and details. This step saves everyone precious time during the appointment and spares you the frustration of re-calling every detail for every question.

Don't let this multiple quizzing frustrate you. There's a method to the madness of three differ-ent people asking you the same question—usually some form of "Why have you come to see the doctor?" They know that the second or third time a patient answers that question, he may provide additional information without even realizing it.

Many doctors send a questionnaire to help patients gather essential information about themselves and their medical histories. Even if you don't receive such a document, be prepared for your doctor's questions by writing down the following information and taking it with you to your initial exam:

- Patient's legal (full) name and maiden name

- Date of birth

- Birthplace

- Parents' names with dates and causes of death

- Current prescribed (Rx) medications, dosing routine, and purpose (example: diazide, 10mg 1 x day for hypertension); list each Rx separately

- Current over-the-counter (OTC) medications taken regularly, including vitamins, supplements, and such (example: calcium+D, 600 mg 2 x day); list each separately

- Any medications (Rx or OTC) taken over the past year but not currently taken

- Known allergies or adverse reactions to medications or common medical equipment (example: latex gloves)

- Other physicians seen regularly (example: allergist, cardiologist)—name, address, telephone

- Current health problems and dates of onset

- Dates and circumstances of past illnesses or medical events (example: fractured rib, heart attack, accident)

- Dates and reasons for hospitalizations

- Dates and reasons for surgeries

- Recent changes in physical health

- Recent changes in mental or emotional health

- Current situations that may contribute to health changes (consider family, work, and other factors)

Stepping through your initial exam

Okay, you have everything in order and today's the appointment. Take some-one with you. If you think you have PD (and it turns out that your doctor agrees), you'll need that extra set of ears to hear what you're bound to miss after you hear that you may have a chronic and progressive condition. Most likely, this will be your care partner if the diagnosis turns out to be PD. The role of this person is to take notes and listen during the appointment and then help you digest and decipher that discussion after the appointment.

Much of what happens at the doctor's office is already familiar to you: the wait (complete with dog-eared selections of last year's magazines); the weigh-in, blood pressure and updating of your medical history; the second wait (this time in the exam room). Use this time to go over the information and questions you've prepared. The doctor's going to ask why you think you have PD, and you need to be prepared to offer specifics (your symptoms, when and how often they occur, when they began, what seems to relieve them, and so on). If you've made a list, you're ready and can just review it.

The doctor may be giving you extra time for your appointment, but that's not the same as endless time. You need to use the time you have wisely by coming to the appointment as well prepared as possible. For more tips on knowing what to expect from a diagnostic appointment and getting the most from that appointment, see "Working with Your Neurologist to Determine Whether This Is PD" section later in this chapter.

Leaving with the answers you need

You'll probably have a gazillion questions by the end of the initial appointment, and you're just as likely not to be able to think of a single one. So once again, be prepared. Prepare a list of questions in advance and use that list. You may even want to hand a copy to your doctor.

If you've brought another person with you to listen and take notes, this is the time she may want to speak up and ask questions also. You can use the following sets of questions as a guide during the appointment. But feel free to add your own.

If the diagnosis seems pretty clear from the start
Although your PCP may believe the diagnosis is clear, he most likely will deliver the news as *possibly* or *likely* Parkinson's and recommend you see a neurologist (a specialist in disorders of the central nervous system). Your PCP may talk in lingo that's unfamiliar to you (*parkinsonism, bradykinesia, postural instability,* and such). Don't be afraid to ask for a clear, layperson's explanation by asking the following questions:

- What is the diagnosis—in plain English?

- What is the prognosis (how quickly will the condition progress)?

- How will the diagnosis be confirmed?

- Does this diagnosis require me to see a specialist?

- Can you recommend a specialist and help set an appointment for me?

- In the meantime, what should I do?

If the doctor orders tests
Even if your doctor believes the diagnosis is fairly clear, she may want to rule out other possibilities. For example, some of the medications you've been taking may be interacting in a way that produces a slight shaking (tremor) in your hand. Or, maybe your primary symptom seems to be depression and apathy; the doctor may want to refer you to a psychologist for evaluation. If she recommends these or other tests, ask the following questions:

- What are the tests and why are you ordering them?

- What is the procedure for each test?

- How quickly will you have the results?

- What will be the next steps after you have the test results?

If the PCP recommends treatment

Especially if you live in a small community or rural area, your PCP may be the only name in town for treating a wide variety of complex conditions. Even if you live in a larger community that has several specialists including neurologists, your doctor may be aware that your economic situation and lack of adequate insurance may keep you from seeking these services. In any case, if your PCP does not recommend seeking a specialist as a next step but does recommend a plan of treatment, ask the following questions:

- What is the treatment?

- Why are you choosing this treatment option?

- What are the risks or possible down sides of taking these medicines or following the recommended therapies?

- What is the cost and will this be covered by my insurance?

- What are the benefits?

- How quickly should the treatment work?

- How will you monitor and follow up on the treatment plan?

- What are the alternatives to this treatment plan?

If It Looks Like PD ... Connecting with a Neurologist

The initial suspicions of you and your PCP will likely lead to an appointment with a neurologist who can administer further tests to confirm the diagnosis. (If your PCP has already diagnosed PD, then your neurologist helps manage your care.) The following sections suggest how to find a specialist in your area and how to know whether you'll make a good team.

Locating an experienced and qualified neurologist

If possible, look for a neurologist who specializes in movement disorders (like Parkinson's). If you're very fortunate, you live in or near a community that has a Morris K. Udall Parkinson's Disease Research Center of Excellence program. These programs—often in a medical university or institution—are involved in clinical research specifically for the benefit of PD patients. (See the "Morris K. Udall Parkinson's Disease Research Centers of Excellence" sidebar for more information.)

This section suggests resources for finding a neurologist who can help you deal with your PD—now and down the road.

Surfing the Web
The Internet can be a huge help to locate a doctor. Several sites locate physicians by specialty as well as by location, and the sites provide important information about a doctor's training, expertise, possible ethical or treatment violations, and so on. Try an online search with the phrase *neurologists finding.*

You can also get information by checking with the local or regional chapter of a national PD organization. (See the next section and Appendix B for the national organization's info.) Ask whether your area has a local PD support group. If it does, ask for the name and contact information of the group's facilitator. When you call the facilitator, ask whether any members of the group have been treated by neurologists that you're considering. If possible, contact those patients (preferably including patients who have changed doctors) and ask about their experiences with those doctors.

Checking with the local chapter of PD groups

The following organizations have chapters and support groups in communities across the country. You can call them to get names of neurologists in your area.

- National Parkinson's Foundation (NPF): 800-327-4545

- American Parkinson's Disease Association (APDA): 800-223-2732

- Parkinson's Action Network (PAN): 800-850-4726

If you live in a small community, you may have to connect with the group in a larger community nearby (or even at the state level), but the information from these experienced groups is invaluable as you look for a neurologist that's right for you.

Asking your family doctor

Your PCP may be an internist or, if you live in a small community or rural area with limited access to medical care, he may be a general practitioner. For some women, an Obstetrician/Gynecologist (OB/GYN) is their PCP. Whatever your doctor's focus, he's probably aware of local leading doctors in various specialties.

A key question to ask your PCP is: Which specialist do you recommend for working in tandem with you (the PCP) and me to manage my overall health and PD? This question is important for many reasons, but mainly because it is enormously important that your neurologist be consulted before any other doctor prescribes medications or treatment that may adversely affect your PD medication routine or worsen your symptoms.

When your town has no neurologists

Speaking of small communities, what are your options if the closest neurologist is some distance away? First, consider that you're not going to see this specialist weekly or even monthly after the diagnosis is confirmed and you begin routine treatment. Second, assuming the neurologist and your PCP are willing to work together, you have the emergency backup of your PCP if you need immediate attention.

Don't be tempted to just let your PCP manage your PD for the sake of convenience. At the very least, you want to have your neurologist reevaluate your treatment and status two to four times a year depending on how much change you experience between visits. If you have questions between appointments, try the phone and e-mail. But, taking a day every two to three months to see the neurologist—the specialist in treating your PD—is time well spent. You're worth every minute of it!

Evaluating your neurologist

First things first. You can't expect a neurologist to cure you because a cure for PD doesn't exist—yet. But you can and should expect a professional partnership. You and your neurologist (as well as other team members that we introduce in Chapter 6) will work together to manage your PD symptoms and maintain your physical, mental, and emotional health to the highest possible levels during the years ahead.

You're looking for a specialist who seems curious about *your* Parkinson's:

- How it's affecting you now

- How you can manage those symptoms best

94

- How to postpone onset of new or worsening symptoms for as long as possible

Morris K. Udall Parkinson's Disease Research Centers of Excellence

Morris K. Udall served in the United States Congress for 30 years and was well-respected by colleagues on both sides of the aisle. He also lived with Parkinson's disease from his diagnosis in 1979 until his death in 1998, serving in the House of Representatives until 1991. In 1997, Congress passed the Morris K. Udall Parkinson's Disease Research Act, and President Clinton signed it into law in 1998. This legislation contributed to the establishment of 12 Parkinson's research centers funded by the National Institute of Neurological Disorders and Stroke (NINDS), a division of the National Institutes of Health (NIH). As a result, the legislation cast a national spotlight on the need for collaborative, coordinated research efforts for new treatments and a cure for PD.

The 12 centers are:

- Brigham and Women's Hospital, Boston, MA

- Columbia University, New York, NY

- Duke University, Durham, NC

- Harvard University (McLean Hospital), Belmont, MA

- Johns Hopkins University, Baltimore, MD

- Massachusetts General Hospital (Massachusetts Institute of Technology), Boston, MA

- Mayo Clinic, Jacksonville, FL

- Northwestern University, Evanston, IL

- University of California Los Angeles (UCLA), Los Angeles, CA

- University of Kentucky Medical Center, Lexington, KY

- University of Virginia, Charlottesville, VA

- University of Pittsburgh, Pittsburgh, PA

The 1997 legislation was a good start, but more work is needed. In 2005, Congressman Lane Evans of Illinois, who also has PD, introduced H.R. 3550, a bill to amend and further the work of the original legislation. The new bill would require NIH to hold a conference to review the progress of the work at these Centers for Excellence every two years and produce a strategic plan (including a budget, expected results, actual spending, and actual results) and a report to Congress. H.R. 3550 was referred to a subcommittee in August of 2005. As of this writing, that was the last action on the bill. The Parkinson's Action Network (PAN) maintains a watch on this bill and other legislation critical to the fight. The Web site is www.parkinsonsaction.org.

Along with expertise, you're looking for a certain quality of empathy—a chemistry between the two of you. (See more discussion on this relationship in the next section.) You don't want a godlike figure that makes decisions *for* you rather than *with* you. After all, who has to live with this PD? Not the neurologist.

Preparing for that first visit

Use the following checklist as you prepare for meeting the neurologist:

- When you make the appointment, ask for the first or last appointment of the day. This choice should assure additional time for questions.

- Make sure your PCP has sent copies of your records to the neurologist's office. Assuming that it was your PCP who referred you to the specialist, you may think that the records are transferred automatically. Guess again. You need to stay on top of this transfer and follow up with both offices to make sure the transfer actually takes place.

- Take a copy of your personal medical history and the results of any recent lab work with you. (Refer back to the section "Preparing for your initial exam" earlier in this chapter for more about the history.)

- Be sure to update that history to include your medications with the strength and dosage routine (or pack up the actual meds in a plastic bag—seriously!). Also list any vitamins, supplements, or other OTC meds you take on a regular basis.

- A few days prior to the appointment, call the office to confirm the appointment and ask whether they've received your records. If they haven't, follow up with your PCP. You may need to pick up copies of the records and take them with you to the appointment.

- Arrive half an hour before your scheduled appointment so you can complete their paperwork without cutting into your time with the doctor.

Interviewing the good doctor

Everyone wants the best neurologist out there. But, because of PD's chronic and progressive nature, you also need a neurologist who's a good fit for you and your care partner. Start with the basic nuts and bolts. The following list contains the most essential factors you need consider:

• Of course the neurologist has a medical degree, but is he *board-certified* (has he completed and passed nationally recognized exams to test his expertise)? If he has special training in *movement disorders* (PD is one), count yourself ahead of the game.

• What professional organizations and societies does he belong to?

• How many people with Parkinson's (PWP) are currently under his care?

• How long has the doctor been treating PWP? (If the good doctor is a good *older* doctor, how long does he anticipate practicing?) If the doctor is relatively young, check background and experience. Has this person worked with more experienced PD specialists?

• Who are the partners in his practice, and what are their backgrounds? No partners? Where does he send patients when he's unavailable?

• What days and hours does he see patients? (If the doctor is well known and sought after but has really limited office hours, that situation may send up a red flag for getting appointments when you need them.)

• Are the office hours and location convenient for you? If not, is that a deal breaker for you? Keep in mind that in the early stages of your PD (see Chapter 3) you'll probably see your neurologist infrequently, perhaps every six to eight weeks. If the distance and schedule still seem inconvenient, you can look elsewhere, but please try not to sacrifice experience and skill for convenience.

• If the doctor orders lab work, does his office provide the service? If not, is the office part of a hospital-physician complex where labs are easily available? If the answer is "No" to both questions, you'll most likely go to your area hospital or walk-in clinic for the lab work.

• What's the cost of an office visit?

• If you need to consult with him by phone, does he charge you for it?

• Does he accept your insurance? If you're on Medicare, does he *accept assignment* (charge only what Medicare assigns as the cost)? See Chapter 20 for more help on those sticky insurance questions.

Reviewing your first impressions

Okay, the neurologist passes your basic tests. Now for the tough part: How well will the two of you work together? First impressions can say a great deal, so pay attention to details like the following:

• Does the doctor seem rushed or distracted when she meets you?

• Does she listen and ask questions that draw out additional information, or does she cut you off making pronouncements rather than recommendations?

• What is her treatment philosophy on PD? Medication right away? Medication only after symptoms start to interfere with life routines? What about the use of new or proven surgical procedures?

The right answer, of course, includes a reminder that all patients progress differently and under varying circumstances, so the treatment regimen varies person to person.

• What is the doctor's philosophy about partnering with the patient (and eventually, when your care partner becomes your advocate and spokesperson, with the care partner)?

• Is there chemistry (we're not talking magic here, just good vibes)? Do you feel an intangible connection—where you can rely on this doctor's partnership to explore ways to manage symptoms and maintain functionality as long as possible?

Moving forward if it's a good fit

Finally, if this doctor seems a good fit, you have just a few more questions to ask him:

• How does the doctor prefer that you prepare for an appointment? For example, does he want you to e-mail questions or concerns in advance, or can you bring written questions to the appointment?

Can you bring a tape recorder to tape the conversation so you can listen to it again?

- What is his preferred way of communicating with you between appointments: by phone or e-mail; through his nurse or physician assistant? (If you're to contact the nurse or physician assistant, be sure you meet this person and get direct contact information.)

- What hospital does the doctor use for treating patients?

And what if, after all of this, the doctor just isn't for you? No chemistry. Of course, you can move on and start the whole process with another doctor. On the other hand, if this doctor is considered the best in your area, perhaps you should give the relationship a chance. After all, the two of you are relative strangers. How well did you click with other professionals in your life on the first appointment? Keep in mind that this is first and foremost a professional relationship; you will rely on this expert to plot the course you'll navigate through the challenges of PD. This doctor may not be especially interested in seeing pictures of your first grandchild, but if the treatment plan he puts together clearly focuses on your individual journey through PD and helps you enjoy that grandchild for years to come, do you really need anything more?

Working with Your Neurologist to Determine Whether This Is PD

Neurologists use a variety of methods to make a definitive diagnosis of PD:

- The physical examination

- An assessment of your function through mental and performance testing

- Sophisticated imaging equipment that permits a look inside your brain

Despite all these methods, your doctor may still need to rule out other explanations for your symptoms before she's prepared to state, without question, that you have PD.

This section takes you through the usual steps of that first visit.

Navigating the clinical exam

No single diagnostic test (like doctors have for measuring blood pressure or cholesterol levels) can confirm a clinical diagnosis of Parkinson's disease. So your neurologist's skill of observation and his experience in diagnosing and treating PWP is key. Your initial appointment will probably include the following three levels of examination:

History taking

The first level of examination is a discussion of your complete medical history. The printed copy you provide (see "Compiling your medical history" earlier in this chapter for help with this step) can help, but you'll probably hear some questions two or three times in this first appointment. Be a *patient* patient (pun intended). A good neurologist asks these questions not only to review your symptoms but also to rule out less-typical types of parkinsonism or other neurological conditions, which sometimes entail radically different management. (See "Parkinsonism, But Not PD" later in this chapter.)

Physical exam

After recording your medical history, the doctor performs a physical examination that may include such standards as:

- Measuring your blood pressure (while you're lying down and then again standing up)

- Checking your pulses, heartbeat, lungs, and abdomen

The point of such routine observations is to make sure your symptoms aren't due to problems in other parts of your body.

Neurological exam
The final level is the neurological examination, which is largely a process of observation. The neurologist tests your coordination and balance while observing you walk, stand, sit, turn, extend your arms and hands, and so on.

This exam may also include any of the following tasks:

- Opening and closing your fists or tapping your fingers several times

- Touching the doctor's finger and then your nose with your index finger (it looks silly but can give the neurologist a wealth of information)

- Recovering your balance after the doctor pulls you gently from behind your shoulders as you stand with your eyes open or closed

- Answering several simple questions from the doctor to test your attention and memory

- Drawing a figure on a piece of paper and then duplicating it

Don't be surprised by the apparent simplicity of these questions and tests; they are all part of a standardized exam!

After the neurologist has completed the initial interview, the physical exam and neurological observations, he (or an assistant) may use standard screening tools to further confirm the diagnosis or the stage or severity of your PD. This next section covers those tools.

Establishing the severity and staging the progression of your PD

Your neurologist may use a variety of tools for establishing your PD's progression through the various stages or levels. (See Chapter 3 for more about these stages.) The rating scales in the next section are useful in setting a benchmark for the doctor. Neuroimaging tools are also helpful in tracking progression and ruling out other possibilities for symptoms you may experience.

Rating scales and neuroimaging tests are tools available to your doctor to assist in establishing the progression of your PDC. They aren't used in confirming the diagnosis.

Rating scales

In any major disorder like PD, neurologists may use standardized rating scales to measure symptoms and stage the disease. (For a refresher on *staging*, flip over to Chapter 3.) These instruments are helpful in determining how advanced your symptoms are and how best to address them. The scales also form the basis for a more extensive medical history if a patient needs to change doctors in the future. In addition, clinical researchers frequently use these scales to monitor the effects of new and experimental therapies on patients. (See Chapter 14, where we discuss the trials more completely.)

• **Hoehn and Yahr Rating Scale:** This diagnostic tool stages the level of a person's PD by using broad measures of disability. This scale was originally devised by Melvin Yahr and Margaret Hoehn following a detailed study of the natural progression of PD in the late 1960s. They observed five general stages in PD, ranging from Stage 1 (unilateral disease, limited to one side of the body) to Stage 5 (wheelchair bound or bedridden unless aided). However, as we mention often in this book, PD doesn't progress in neat, little, predictable stages. Therefore, the more complex (and more informative) Unified Parkinson Disease Rating Scale (see the next section) usually accompanies and complements this tool.

• **Unified Parkinson Disease Rating Scale (UP-DRS):** The UPDRS focuses on several facets of PD's disability, such as its effects on daily activities, motor skills, and mental capacity (including behavior and mood). It consists of a painless interview and a focused neurological exam, with a score for each item from 0 (normal) to 4 (severe). Therefore, the higher the UPDRS score, the greater the disability from PD.

The UPDRS—when administered correctly—is "an exquisitely sensitive test for detecting early PD," according to a Parkinson's Disease Foundation article. It may be the best tool for the neurologist to assess symptom levels and design treatment plans. The UPDRS is currently under revision by the Movement Disorders Society and will be soon updated to better reflect the multifaceted reality of PD disability.

• **Schwab and England Activities of Daily Living:** This tool rates a person's ability to perform the normal routine activities of daily living using a percentage rating. The patient usually rates himself with the help of set definitions presented by the doctor.

For example, people who consider themselves to be completely independent and functional qualify for a 100 percent rating. They can perform all activities without difficulty. In contrast, a person who takes three to four times the normal time to perform a task (such as dressing) has a 70 percent independence rating. And a person who can manage only a few chores from time to time (and always with great effort) has a 30 percent rating.

Neuroimaging
A thorough neurological exam and the proper administration of the UPDRS is usually enough to diagnose a new case of PD. However, neuroimaging techniques now permit neurologists to pinpoint the diagnosis of PD and follow its progression by observing the affected nerve cells.

Two recently developed imaging techniques, positron-emission tomography and single photon emission computed tomography, can confirm the diagnosis of PD and distinguish PD from other Parkinson-like disorders. (See "Parkinsonism, But Not PD" later in this chapter for more discussion on other disorders.) Both scans use low levels of radioactive materials and pose little, if any, risk for the patient. I describe both of these scans in the following:

* The *positron-emission tomography* (PET) scan uses a radioactive form of *levodopa* (the drug that en-

110

hances dopamine production in the brain), which is injected intravenously into the patient, to highlight the loss of normal *dopamine* cells (the neurons primarily affected by PD) in the brain. As dopamine cells uptake levodopa, a reduced signal from labeled (radioactive) levodopa is usually found in PD.

- The *single photon emission computed tomography* (SPECT) scan is another imaging technique able to measure metabolic and physiological functions of specific areas of the brain. When using radioactive markers able to link to dopamine cells, SPECT scans can measure the progressive loss of these neurons caused by PD.

A couple of factors limit the use of neuroimaging: cost and availability. At this writing, some insurance companies consider such scans experimental and as a result, don't cover any of the costs. In addition, the equipment and expertise for performing and interpreting the scans aren't widely available.

Ruling out the red herrings: What else can it be?

What else looks like PD? That answer may depend on your presenting symptoms (the information you tell the doctor) or on other facts that the doctor gathers through interviewing and examining you.

For example:

- If you don't present with any of the *TRAP* symptoms (check out Chapter 3 for a quick review of these) but you talk about a loss of energy, the doctor may want to explore that symptom more. After further questioning, your doctor may see that depression plays a role in your loss of energy. If so, is the depression associated with PD, or is it related to some other life-changing event, such as the death of a loved one or the loss of a job?

- Even if a hand tremor was your reason for seeing a neurologist, is the tremor confined to one hand or both? Does it stop after the hand is engaged in activity, or does the tremor continue?

Don't try to second-guess your symptoms. Is it PD? Maybe. Is it something else—something easier to treat and cure? Possibly. Either way, you need to know. Why postpone treating a curable condition simply because you think it may be more serious? And if it does turn out to be PD, then you want to get a jump on managing symptoms as early as possible—when you have the greatest opportunity to maintain independence and flexibility.

Parkinsonism, But Not PD

If it walks like a duck and quacks like a duck, it's a duck, right? So if it looks like PD and acts likes PD, then it's PD, right? Not always.

The same symptoms that indicate PD can also indicate other conditions, thus *parkinsonism* is a generic term referring to slowness and mobility problems that look like PD. Parkinsonism is a feature in several conditions that have different (and perhaps known) causes, but those conditions don't progress like PD. As a result, years may go by before the differences between PD and the other disorder are apparent; the PD diagnosis may then be reversed.

Taking antiparkinsonian medications (such as levodopa) may be the first indicator that parkinsonism isn't actually PD. By definition, PD promptly responds to this medication, which improves its symptoms in a consistent way, at least for a few years. But, in parkinsonism, improvement is often erratic or nonexistent from the beginning. In fact, your neurologist will always closely monitor your response to treatment in order to rule out the possibility that your condition is a disorder other than PD.

Two categories of non-PD disorders are:

- **Parkinson's Plus syndromes:** This group of neurodegenerative disorders has parkinsonian features, such as *bradykinesia* (slowness), *rigidity* (stiffness), *tremor* (shaking), and *gait disturbances* (balance). See Chapter 3 for more about these PD symptoms. However, they are also associated with other complex neurological symptoms that reflect problems in brain areas other than the *dopaminergic system* (the network of neurons able to make and release the neurotransmitter *dopamine*). These conditions progress more rapidly than PD and don't respond as well (or at all) to antiparkinsonian medications. The most common Parkinson's Plus syndromes are *Multiple System Atrophy* (MSA), *Progressive Supranuclear Palsy* (PSP), *Cortico-Basal Ganglion-*

114

ic Degeneration (CBGD), and *Lewy Body Dementia* (LBD).

- **Secondary parkinsonisms:** The symptoms of these disorders relate to well-defined lesions in the brain from strokes, tumors, infections, traumas, or certain drugs. Like Parkinson's Plus syndromes, these syndromes are usually less responsive to levodopa. However, if the primary cause of parkinsonism is controlled, these symptoms tend to be less progressive.

In addition to Parkinson's plus and secondary parkinsonisms, *Essential Tremor* (ET) is another source of possible confusion. As the most common movement disorder—as much as 20 times more common than PD—ET's only symptom is a tremor that affects the hands (only while they're moving) but may also affect the head or voice. ET can run in families and is usually benign and non-disabling. The much-admired actress, Katherine Hepburn, may have suffered from ET—not PD.

This Is Your Life—Getting a Second (or Even Third) Opinion

Whatever the diagnosis, if you have concerns, questions, or doubts, then you have every reason to get a second or even a third opinion. After all, you know your body and its symptoms better than anyone else.

So if you live within a reasonable distance of a Udall Center (see the sidebar "Morris K. Udall Parkinson's Disease Research Centers of Excellence" earlier in this chapter) or a medical center with a reputation for excellent PD care and research, see whether you can get an appointment and check out what those folks say. Even if you have to travel some distance, the information will be worth the trip.

Another reason to seek a second or third opinion is to find a neurologist you have chemistry with. The doctor who delivered the initial diagnosis may be a fine neurologist with great credentials and experience, but maybe the two of you had no connection and you don't see a partnership with her. With PD, you don't want to be switching from one doctor to another. So, find a doctor that you can build a real partnership with now—one with a proactive and optimistic philosophy about meeting the challenges of living with PD.

The danger lies in seeking one opinion after another just because you didn't like the first (or second or third) answer—even though, in your heart-of-hearts, you're sure it's true. That's called *denial.* Because you may not want to face the future, you keep running after more opinions, hoping some day some doctor will say you don't have PD.

After a doctor has confirmed the diagnosis (and perhaps another doctor has reconfirmed it), you need to accept it and prepare yourself and your family for the journey. Maybe you've already made significant progress by finding a neurologist that you and your PCP can partner with to maintain and manage your health for the long term.

Chapter 5

You've Been Diagnosed—Now What?

In This Chapter

• Facing your fears about Parkinson's disease

• Establishing your long-term vision and short-term goals

• Caring for the future: Advice for your partner

Okay, it's official—you have Parkinson's disease (PD). In these first days following that blow, no doubt your emotions are rocketing. And like a pinball, they're bouncing moment to moment and hour to hour around those Five Stages of Grief that Elisabeth Kubler-Ross introduced:

• Can't be (denial)

• Shouldn't be (anger)

• Don't let it be (bargaining)

- Why me? (depression)

- IS! (acceptance or at least realization)

A sixth stage to consider in facing a diagnosis of PD is *hope.* You can find some measure of control as you continue toward the future you had already planned—one that did *not* include living with a chronic and progressive illness.

And that's the purpose of this chapter—to help you move beyond those first jumbled emotions of diagnosis toward a clearly focused, take-charge attitude of this disease. In this chapter we first talk you through the emotional steps and then guide you toward healthy goals and plans for coming to grips with PD. We also address your care partner, the one who plans to walk that walk with you, and offer advice for these early months after the diagnosis.

Sorting Out Your Emotions

Depending on your past awareness or experiences with PD, either you have some idea of how your life is going to change or you have no idea at all. In either case, your imagination can get carried away with all the what-ifs.

Stop! This is a new challenge, but it's not so different from other challenges that have taken your life in unexpected directions. Every day people face un-planned events that change the course they thought they were on—job losses, break-ups in relationships, unplanned moves to different locations, the loss of a loved one, hurricanes, and floods. Life happens.

Take a breath. Any challenges that you faced (and survived) in the past (like raising your children, building your career, caring for aging parents, and such) gave you key building blocks and tools to face this new challenge.

Now, give yourself time to:

- Understand that a PD diagnosis is not a death sentence. You have a life to live and choices to make about how you'll face each day, probably for years and even decades to come.

- Believe that past experiences have given you the tools you need to cope with PD.

- Accept the difference between what you can and can't control. Focus on what you can.

- Connect with people who are positive and upbeat.

- Banish negative self-talk ("I can't," or "I won't," and such), and turn the negative to a positive ("I can" and "I will").

- Embrace the joys in your life—your partner, children, friends, work or avocation, love of music, art, sports, and so on.

- Help yourself by helping other people—volunteer, get involved, make a difference.

- Recognize the opportunities you have to educate others, advocate for change (and a cure), make new friends, and know your deeper self.

Basically you have two choices: Define your life as a person with Parkinson's (PWP) or live that life to the fullest—the same as if you'd never been diagnosed with PD.

Dodging denial and meeting your diagnosis head on

When you get the confirmed diagnosis, you and your family—especially your partner—need time to digest the news and react. And the first reaction for one or both of you may be denial. Your partner may become overprotective and treat you as if you're gravely ill. Financial concerns may pop up; your partner may wonder about the costs and sacrifices. Underneath your partner may first feel cheated out of the life you had planned and then angry at such a selfish thought when you're facing a debilitating illness. (For more help in dealing with such difficult feelings, see Chapter 22.)

Neither you nor your partner may admit any of these feelings initially. Big mistake. Your fastest route to coping is to work through such feelings together by openly communicating your fears and concerns and then working through possible solutions to each. Following the guidelines set forth in the remainder of this chapter can help.

Denial can take two forms. First, many people who receive the diagnosis of PD—or any other serious illness—soon realize that the early symptoms have been there. Perhaps you dismissed those early warning signs for weeks or even months because you were afraid or didn't want other people to know you had some troublesome symptoms.

The second form of denial comes after you've received the diagnosis. Now the facts are out there. You're human, and no doubt the actual news that you have PD has come as a real blow. *Initially* refusing to believe this is happening is your mind's way of giving you time to gather the necessary strength to go forward.

However, *sustaining* that denial takes an enormous amount of energy—energy that can be much more valuable in facing the actual challenge. Refusing to acknowledge the truth means you're forcing yourself to keep a secret from other people and yourself.

In spite of your denial, deep inside you know this diagnosis is real. You may even be surprised to realize you have a slight feeling of relief because the enemy has a name, and now you can begin to fight it. You can't go back and not have PD. But you can decide how best to move forward.

Allowing yourself to get angry

Anger is an understandable reaction to news like this. The question is: Who's on the receiving end of that anger? The world in general? Your friends and family who've never taken care of themselves like you always have? Your significant other (who you fear—in your current, warped state of mind—may leave you)? God? How about yourself?

Go ahead—rant, rave, and howl at the moon. A little healthy anger is good for you, and certainly you deserve to indulge that anger—within reason. Try these tips for giving anger your best shot.

- Keep the focus on the object of your anger—having PD. It's easier than you may suspect to broaden that focus until suddenly everything and everyone makes you mad.

- Start figuring out ways you're going to get back at this enemy that's attacked your perfectly good life (the same way you'd think of ways to get back at the boss who passed you over for that promotion). For example, you can say to your Parkinson's, "I'll show you that I can still lead my life in spite of the challenges you throw my way!"

- Set limits. When you're overwhelmed by your fury at the unfairness of this diagnosis, set a kitchen timer for 10 minutes. When the bell dings, you're done—at least for today.

- Find the humor—black though it may be—in this unexpected and unwanted situation and defuse your anger with that humor.

Anger (like denial and a bunch of other normal reactions to news of a chronic, progressive illness) is non-productive *unless* it leads you to fight back. Permit yourself some time to work your way through this news. (For some people, this will be a matter of days; for others it's a couple of weeks.) If the feelings continue longer than that, you need to get some help to resolve the anger. Throughout the course of your PD, you're going to be upset and angry from time to time. Your goal is not to dwell in that anger but to transform its energy into determination to regain control and move forward.

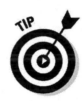

Admitting you're scared

Chances are good that you still don't have a handle on the full impact of this diagnosis. Getting your head around the concept of a lifelong, progressive illness is a pretty tall order, especially in the beginning. It's enough to scare the bejeebers out of anyone! You have so many questions and fears. How do you deal with them?

There's no shame in admitting you're scared. The title song from the musical *Cabaret* says, "Start by admitting from cradle to grave, it isn't that long a stay." In other words, life is what we get—no promises and no guarantees. The unknown can be intriguing, exhilarating, or frightening. And certainly, when that unknown is PD, you may find yourself even feeding that fear through your responses to it.

Instead of further terrifying yourself by reading every case study, article, or book you can get your hands on about PD, place limits on how much information you need and can handle—especially at the beginning. Instead of smiling politely as some well-meaning clerk or neighbor relates his horror story about a fifth-cousin-twice-removed who had PD back in the dark ages, thank him for his concern and leave. Instead of allowing other people to educate you based on hearsay, observations from afar, and an article they read about former Attorney General Janet Reno, educate yourself.

Using the reputable and frequently updated resources listed in Appendix B, you can gather the information you need to become the true expert on what is and isn't possible with PD. Then, when people start telling you about your condition and how to manage your life, quietly but firmly correct them. Trust us; nothing silences a know-it-all like someone who really does know. And nothing helps you get a handle on that gut-wrenching fear like educating yourself on the realities, possibilities, and opportunities for expanding your life—of living with PD.

Getting to acceptance

No one is denying that you need to work through a whole range of emotions, but you can't stay locked in those emotional prisons. When you move through them, you free yourself to fully live your days.

You have a chronic and progressive illness, but

- You have years ahead of you.

- You're still productive.

- You have time to pursue dreams and goals.

- You can live life on your terms if you accommodate PD as *part* of that life, not *all* of it.

How to go about that? Start with these key steps:

- Get the best treatment you can after you have the diagnosis. Part III of this book is all about treatment options, some that you may find surprisingly easy to incorporate into your life.

- Deal with the emotional roller coaster of living with a chronic progressive illness. Chapters 13 and 22 offer tips on facing the depression, anxiety, and other difficult feelings that are part and parcel of living with any chronic progressive conditions.

- Manage your inevitable lifestyle changes and social adjustments with family and friends (and theirs with you). Check out Chapter 7 for tips on who, how, and when to tell about your PD; then look at Chapter 15 for more in-depth advice on maintaining key relationships.

- Protect your unique sense of self-worth and identity. Well, we could just remind you to read this whole book because our key message in every chapter is that you can live with this condition. In fact, you can have a full and satisfying life—it just won't be the life you thought you were going to have (but isn't that true for most people?).

Sometimes acceptance comes most easily when you turn your attention to the people who love you and have heard your diagnosis. They're wrestling with high anxiety too. Of course, their first concern is for you, but a part of that concern is PD's effect on their relationship with you. How will their lives change with yours? When you acknowledge their fears (as well as your own) and explore that with them, you create an environment of "we're in this thing together" that goes a long way toward sustaining everyone when times get tough. (Tips for ways you can best communicate with other people are in Chapters 7 and 15.)

By taking the lead in figuring out how to live with PD, in many ways you become a mentor. You're the person others look to and trust to show the best way to face this life-changing situation. For many of us, actor Christopher Reeve and his wife, Dana, were the poster couple for finding grace in the face of unspeakable adversity. Think about it: If you built your career as *Superman* and ended up unable to move much less leap over tall buildings, wouldn't you be tempted to feel sorry for yourself? Instead Christopher Reeve found the will and the courage to use his adversity to inspire and motivate people and make a real difference in the world.

No one expects you to become a national icon now that you have PD. But you can become that mentor for people closest to you. Through your attitude and approach, you can set the tone for the way others interact with you and incorporate PD into the relationship.

Taking charge and moving forward

Prepare but don't project needs to be your mantra. The temptation to look ahead and worry about the future can be overwhelming. Our advice: Fight that instinct! Given a diagnosis of a chronic and progressive disease that has no cure, a person's natural tendency is to try and foretell the future. Major mistake!

With PD, every patient's journey is unique, so projecting what may happen can only increase your anxiety. You and your care partner can go crazy, racing around and trying to cover all your possible challenges even before they develop.

The point is that you have a disease that will require—like most health conditions—changes to your lifestyle. For example,

• What will you do if you can no longer manage the stairs in your current home, but the bedrooms (and the main bathroom) are all upstairs?

In Chapter 21, we explore many options for staying in your current residence in spite of obstacles such as this. For example, you may have a room on the first floor that you can adapt as a bedroom; maybe you can convert a half-bath into a full bathroom (with the addition of a shower); or your stairway may be wide enough to accommodate an electric chair lift.

• As your ability to move decreases, how will you handle an emergency such as getting out of the house in the event of a fire?

Even if you didn't have PD, common sense should move every family to have an emergency plan in place. So sit down with the family and figure this one out—for you and everyone else in the household. One solution is to talk to people at your local fire and police department and get their suggestions.

Our guess is that throughout your life (and certainly as an adult) you've planned for the possibility of unexpected changes or events. And even though those plans may come in a year or not at all, you've still considered the options and are prepared to act.

Taking Action

Think of PD as a 400-pound lineman constantly in your face. He's there when you wake up and when you go to sleep. He gets in your way, blocking you when you try to work or play and when your friends come around. Sometimes he's well-behaved, maybe even sitting on the sidelines for a while. But mostly he's charging, blocking, and even tackling to keep you from doing what you want.

How do you get around this lineman? The answer is that sometimes you won't. But other times—most of the time—you can find new and innovative ways to live life on your terms. Managing a chronic illness means you need to give up control over some parts of your life and take control in new ways. Some of those new controls are:

• Educating yourself and your family about your PD

• Developing a long-range strategy for managing your PD

• Turning negatives into positives through creative problem-solving

- Being a real team player—with your healthcare team (see Chapter 6), your care partners, and other PWP

Arming yourself with good information

The key to gathering information is making sure it's trustworthy and evidence-based. The Agency for Healthcare and Research (an agency within the Department of Health and Human Services) recommends these resources:

- **healthfinder** (www.healthfinder.gov) is sponsored by the U.S. Department of Health and Human Services. The site includes links to government agencies, clearinghouses, non-profit groups, and universities.

- **Health Information Resource Database** (www.health.gov/nhic/#Referrals or 800-336-4797) is sponsored by the National Health Information Center. This site offers information on more than 1000 organizations and government agencies that provide health information on request.

- **MEDLINEplus** (www.nlm.nih.gov/medlineplus) is sponsored by the National Institutes of Health (NIH). The site has extensive information from NIH and other trusted resources on more than 650 diseases and conditions.

- **Non-profit organizations** such as the National Parkinson's Foundation and The Michael J. Fox Foundation focus specifically on PD. For a complete list and contact information, see Appendix B.

In addition, try checking with medical libraries in your area (but keep in mind that this information is for physicians, medical students, and researchers—the reading can get fairly technical).

Ignore information from

- Product advertisements that

    • Make extraordinary claims, such as *scientific breakthrough* or *secret formula.*

    • Claim to work for a number of different conditions.

    • Claim the product is available from only one source or for a limited time.

- Well-meaning friends who have

> • Heard of some therapy but can't recall the source.
>
> • Had a relative who tried *x-treatment.* It worked for that person, so it's bound to work for you!

• Well-meaning strangers who, in their zeal to show sympathy for your condition, rattle off several ideas about treatment.

Jotting down the questions you have

Chances are good that you were pretty numb as you sat in the doctor's office and received the news. (See Chapter 4, where we cover the initial visit with the neurologist.) But now you realize you have all sorts of questions. Or perhaps you asked questions at the time and your doctor offered information, but you really didn't take it in.

Schedule a second appointment (if you haven't already) and let your doctor (or the nurse) know that you want to be able to ask questions and discuss issues that have come to mind since the diagnosis. At that appointment, bring your list of questions (as well as your care partner for that second set of ears) and be ready to take notes. The following questions are a sampling of some concerns you may want to cover.

- What's the technical name of my condition, and what does that mean in plain English?

- What's the *prognosis,* my outlook for the future?

- How soon do I need to make a decision about treatment?

- Will I need additional tests? If so, what kind and when?

- What are my treatment options, and what are the pros and cons of those treatment options?

- What changes will I need to make in my daily life?

- What resources and organizations do you recommend for support and information?

- What resources can your office provide (books, pamphlets, audio or videotapes, and such) that I can review right away?

- And, the question uppermost in your mind: Am I going to die from this?

Establishing realistic and attainable goals

If PD is to be part of your life but not your entire life, then you need a game plan. Fact: If you don't have a plan for dealing with PD, then it will dominate every facet of your life. This section takes you through specific steps toward making and living that plan.

In the world of business, executive teams meet regularly. Their purpose? To plan for the future success of their business. Their process usually follows a three-step course:

1. **Establish a long-term vision.**

2. **Set short-term goals toward achieving that vision.**

3. **Identify and prioritize tasks necessary to attain those goals.** (This is known as the *Plan of Action,* or POA.)

To apply these three steps to PD, the first step (the vision) is already established: to live a productive and satisfying life for as long as possible in spite of PD.

The second step (setting goals) requires you to set aside sentimentality. As much as people wish otherwise, PD (as of this writing) has no cure. So, a goal of being cured is neither realistic nor attainable. As you consider your real goals, remember the following principles:

- Keep them simple.

- Keep them practical.

- Keep them specific.

The third step is the POA. Did you ever see a milk stool, the three-legged variety farmers sat on to milk cows? That three-legged approach is the way you need to think about your POA over the long term because living with PD is not only a physical challenge; it's also a mental and emotional one. And, just like the milk stool, if one leg is missing, the plan will topple.

The following sections provide examples of three goals and their POAs that support a long-term vision for PD.

Goal 1: Maintain maximum physical function

PD has no magic pill. So, after confirming your diagnosis, your neurologist will probably have a number of recommendations that may include management of symptoms with proven medications, physical and occupational therapy, and perhaps a program for diet and exercise.

Although medications and traditional medical interventions may help minimize your symptoms, you enhance your opportunity to achieve your long-term vision when you maintain your best physical condition. On the other hand, if you ignore the doctor's prescription for changes in your lifestyle (such as adjustments to your diet and activity routines or a specific timetable for taking your medications), you compromise your overall vision. (See Chapter 9 for more about the importance of sticking to your medication schedule and Chapter 12 for a full discussion of exercise and nutrition.)

No one has all of the symptoms. Although PD is a chronic, progressive condition, its path varies tremendously from one person to the next. You are unique—as a person and as a PWP. You and your medical team need to keep that in mind as together you select those options (medications, therapies, and lifestyle changes) that have the greatest effect on maintaining your physical function for as long as possible.

Goal 2: Keep your mind sharp

You're certainly going to have a lot on your mind in the days and weeks to come as you and your medical team put together a viable plan for managing your PD symptoms. And you're going to hear a lot of new words—words that PD specialists, PWPs, and their care partners throw around as easily as *apple* or *orange.*

You can refuse to follow that technical PD jargon (and everything else about this intruder), or you can become an expert, someone who actively seeks out background information about PD, understands and uses the technical lingo, and keeps up with the research and new treatment options.

This advice doesn't mean PD has to become your life's work. You have more important (and fun!) ways to spend your time. But remember: Knowledge is power, and seeking out that knowledge exercises your brain. Get started using the resources listed in Appendix B. Getting a grip on PD (what it is and isn't) is a good place to start—but don't stop there.

What are your interests and how did you challenge your mind before you had PD? Are you a sports enthusiast who enjoys statistics and box scores? Do you enjoy brainteasers, like crossword puzzles, jigsaw puzzles, or word games? Do you love good music, art, and theater?

Continuing to engage your mind in enjoyable ways is as important to your POA as pushing yourself physically. Don't turn your back on the intellectual life you enjoyed before PD.

Goal 3: Embrace the power of emotional and spiritual well-being

Going through a range of emotions post-diagnosis is normal. But anxiety and depression can be viable symptoms of PD as well as viable responses to its diagnosis. Your doctor needs to know if you're experiencing persistent (longer than a couple of weeks) sadness or apathy. (See Chapter 14 for a full discussion of the effects of anxiety and depression in PD.)

Although your neurologist or primary care physician (in consultation with each other) can prescribe medication and professional counseling to help you through these negative emotions, you can also be proactive by

- Acknowledging that these persistent negative feelings are abnormal.

- Finding a support group where you can discuss feelings with other people who

  Perhaps have similar emotions.

  Recognize these emotions as part of the adaptive process in dealing with PD.

- Accepting the support of family and friends as you come to terms with PD and its effects on all your lives.

In concert with your medical team, you can address physical, mental, and even emotional needs as part of your POA. However, one facet of your care plan only you can develop is a plan for your spiritual health. This facet goes beyond faith and religious rituals, although those resources certainly help.

Spiritual health means going inside yourself and coming to terms with your illness day by day. For some PWP, coping comes through challenging activities: participating in sports, continuing to pursue a career, traveling, and so on. If these challenges help you find inner peace and comfort, great!

142

Other PWP may find spiritual healing in quieter pursuits: a walk in the park or along the beach; music; reading; sitting quietly in a secluded, deserted place. These activities are also excellent choices for maintaining spiritual health.

Take care that your solitude doesn't become a regular hiding place to wallow over your losses. Be aware that seclusion can sometimes lead to depression.

Living your life to the fullest

You can perform a lot of actions to fight PD and its effects. But thousands of PWP believe that a huge part of fighting PD is to approach it as only a piece of their lives. The point is this: Those facets of your life that defined you before you were diagnosed are still there—at least for the most part. If you were a parent before, you still are and your child (children) needs you as much as before. If you had a career that you enjoyed (even loved), don't allow PD to become your new, full-time occupation. If you enjoyed sports, music, and other leisure activities, get creative about finding new ways to enjoy those pastimes. In short, LIVE!

The road will be challenging, but as actor and PD advocate, Michael J. Fox, wrote in his biography, *Lucky Man,* "If you were to rush into this room right now and announce that you had struck a deal—with God, Allah, Buddha, Christ, Krishna, Bill Gates, whomever—in which the ten years since my diagnosis could be magically taken away, traded in for the person I was before, I would, without a moment's hesitation, tell you to take a hike."

Next steps

Getting information you can trust so you can form the questions to ask so you can establish some clear goals for managing this condition—pretty tall order! Consider these three concrete steps that you can take right now to get started:

1. Go online and bookmark the sites listed in Appendix B if you have access to a computer.

These national organizations are your best resource for the latest updates on treatments as well as tips for managing your PD symptoms. Get into the habit of regularly checking in on the sites you find most useful. If the site offers an e-list, sign up.

2. Call the toll-free numbers for the PD organizations if you don't have access to a computer.

Ask them to send you their printed materials and add you to the mailing list for new materials in the future.

3. Keep reading.

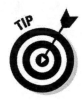

Before you turn to the next chapter, take a moment to read through the following with your family—especially the person who is most likely to be your primary care partner. Even though these sections (scattered throughout this book) are labeled *for the care partner,* try to read them together. The information applies to both of you because you have a responsibility to acknowledge that your care partner has a life beyond helping you manage your PD. (You may also want to check out Chapter 24 for more tips about how to give and receive care and support.)

A Word for the PD Care Partner

In many chronic, progressive illnesses (for example, Alzheimer's disease), family members must increasingly take charge. With PD, however, the PWP can be in charge most of the way. As the care partner, you may want to take over, especially as tasks become more difficult and decisions take longer for your partner to process. But resist that urge. Partnering-in-care is not doing *for*—it's doing *with*.

But where does that leave you as you face your own fears and anxieties about living with someone who has a chronic, progressive condition that won't go away but will color your lives for years to come? Go back and reread this chapter. Everything we suggest for the PWP applies to you as well:

- Sort through your emotions; deal with the anger, the fear, and the realities of how life is going to change (see also Chapter 22).

- Adopt a take charge/move forward/don't look back outlook and start preparing for eventualities that may occur down the road. (You may especially want to read Chapters 20 and 21 about housing options and financial and legal matters.)

- Be proactive. Educate yourself; go to doctor and therapy appointments with the PWP and take notes; become a combination of cheerleader and coach as your loved one faces new challenges.

- Set goals that allow you to maintain a life and identity beyond your role as care partner.

The best support you can offer over the long term is to be a fierce advocate for your loved one's autonomy and independence. The next best way to show support is to take care of yourself and see that your needs are also met. By working together—in partnership—the two of you can take something that could have destroyed you and turn it into a life-experience that enriches you in ways you cannot yet imagine.

Chapter 6

Drafting Your Healthcare Team and a Game Plan

In This Chapter

- Recruiting your professional care team

- Prepping for unexpected scenarios

- Touching base with your care partner

Knowledge may be power, but with today's constant bombardment of information, you need a team of experts that can answer questions and address unexpected situations with the most-advanced procedures.

People with Parkinson's (PWP), like people with other chronic-care needs, must rely on the expertise of several different professionals throughout the course of their illness. In this chapter, professionals and their roles in managing your Parkinson's symptoms are defined. You also take a look at how best to handle hospitalizations, emergency room visits, and other unexpected medical predicaments and complications that are possible for PWP. Last, but not least, your care partner gets ideas for building his own team.

Introducing Your Teammates

Each member of your professional Parkinson's disease (PD) team has special talents and expertise that can help you manage symptoms and maintain normal function and quality of life, often for years following the initial diagnosis. In this section, you discover a list of professionals and their roles in your care, and then you uncover your role in helping these pros perform at their very best.

Lining up the doctors

At least two doctors will help set the course for your care after your PD diagnosis. In addition, you may have other specialists (or you may add them at a later date) if you have other chronic conditions, such as arthritis, hypertension, and the like. The more doctors you have, the more vital it becomes for one doctor (most likely your primary care physician) to take the role of quarterback to oversee and coordinate the plan to meet all your health needs.

Your primary care physician
Your *primary care physician* (PCP) may be a general practitioner (GP) who focuses on family medicine or that person may be an internist who treats adults

only. You've probably been seeing this doctor for some time and have built a trust and style of communication that works for both of you. Now that you have PD, you need to talk with your PCP about two things: his willingness to consult and communicate with your neurologist (who'll take the lead on treating your PD symptoms), and how your PD treatment can integrate with your overall healthcare plan.

Your neurologist

Chances are good that your PCP referred you to a neurologist to confirm the PD diagnosis. If so, these two professionals may already have a good working relationship. However, if you went for a second (or even third) opinion and chose another neurologist to oversee your PD care, be sure that these two doctors meet and show a clear willingness to work together. It's also helpful if your PCP and neurologist are on staff at the same hospital in case you need hospitalization or emergency treatment down the road. (For tips on locating and choosing a neurologist, see Chapter 4.)

Other specialists

In the event you need to consult with other specialists (a cardiologist, urologist, or the like) for new medical situations that arise, these physicians must work closely with your PCP and neurologist so they're all communicating from the same play book (to continue the sports analogy). Think of these doctors as coming off the bench. When they get into the game, they need to get up to speed on your game plan and their specific roles.

Before you keep an appointment with a specialist ask your PCP (and neurologist, if appropriate) to send the specialist(s) a copy of your most recent records. After your visit with one of these doctors, ask that a copy of the office visit report be sent to your PCP with a copy sent to you at the same time. With this exchange of information between doctors—and by assembling your own file of reports—you enhance the likelihood that everyone is on the same page, working from the same information.

Calling up the therapists

Because PD is a movement disorder that affects your ability to perform basic movements, your physical, occupational, and (possibly) speech therapists are very important. These professionals offer proven methods to enhance and pro-long your control of symptoms, and improve your overall sense of well-being. Their services may or may not be covered by insurance unless your doctor's prescription notes them as *medically necessary* to treat your PD.

Physical therapist

A physical therapist (PT) can teach you how to build muscle strength, increase flexibility, and improve co-ordination and balance to prevent falls and serious fractures. Techniques may include exercise programs (standard as well as alternatives, like yoga), heat and cold packs, and water therapy (exercises in water).

Your PT can design a program of exercises specific to your individual symptoms and abilities to preserve and even increase your muscle strength and flexibility.

Although exercise doesn't appear to slow the progression of PD, recent studies indicate that exercise may help prevent the orthopedic muscular and skeletal effects of *akinesia* (slowed or impaired ability to move) and lessen *rigidity* (stiff muscles). Exercise helps you maintain balance and prevent falls.

Your PT can't work miracles. If you only exercise when you go to a session with your PT, you're not likely to see ongoing or long-term benefits. When the physical therapy sessions end (or when the time between sessions stretches to two weeks or more), you need to pursue your own regular program of

152

stretching, strengthening, and aerobic exercises if you want the physical therapy to be successful in the long run. See Chapter 12 for a suggested program of stretches and exercises.

Occupational therapist

Essentially, the *occupational therapist* (OT) helps preserve your sense of independence and self-confidence by showing you new ways of performing simple and routine tasks (known in the medical profession as *activities of daily living* or ADLs) that may have become difficult for you. One significant benefit of working with an OT is simply knowing that you can preserve your control (with alternative techniques) when the loss of control seems a foregone conclusion. For example, she may teach you new techniques (such as a *cueing* or a reminder system) and provide assistive devices (such as a special cane) that help you perform certain movements and tasks.

For more information on ways to adapt to your changing symptoms, check out the information in Part III on living with PD.

Speech therapist

Not every PWP needs speech therapy, but if you're experiencing a softened vocal tone, unintentional mispronunciations, or wrong word choices, a speech therapist can help. These professionals can also help if you ever develop swallowing or other throat muscle problems that can come with PD.

If a trained speech therapist isn't available in your area, consider trying a program especially for PWP called the Lee Silverman Voice Treatment or LSVT. For more information about the LSVT Foundation, its programs, and links to other PD groups, see www.lsvt.org.

Drafting other team players

As a PWP, you have your front-line defense consisting of your PCP, your neurologist, and trained movement and speech therapists. But, have you considered the number of other professionals that can help you to manage your symptoms and continue living a normal life as long as possible? Be sure that you include the following care professionals and experts when you're assembling the team.

Pharmacist

Your pharmacist is in the business of knowing medications and their interactions. She knows your current medications, their potential side effects, and the possible impact of any new medication that your PCP or neurologist may prescribe. And, because this is her area of expertise, she's your best resource for answering your questions after you've carefully read the printed information on your prescriptions. (For more information about prescription medicines, be sure to check out Chapter 9.)

Your job? Pick one pharmacy (or chain that shares information among all branches) to fill all your prescriptions and stick with them. Then be sure the pharmacist knows which over-the-counter (OTC) medicines you're taking or considering taking.

Psychologist or counselor

Anxiety and depression are part and parcel of having PD, and they're perfectly normal reactions to hearing a diagnosis of a chronic, progressive condition. A trained and licensed counselor can be a key member of your professional care team. Whether you see this person on a regular basis for *talk therapy sessions* (see Chapter 13 for more on this topic) or just now and then for some emotional unburdening, go ahead and identify this counselor shortly after your diagnosis is confirmed.

Support groups

Throughout this book we tout the benefits of joining a support group—for you and your care partner. You may reject this idea in the early stages. "I don't want to sit around talking to a bunch of strangers or listening to them complain about their PD. I've got my own problems." Wrong! Well, sort of. You definitely have your own problems. But, here's the point you're missing: A support group can help you find ways to cope with those problems.

Many types of support groups are around for PWP and their care partners. Some groups take a broader advocacy approach, while other groups focus more on their members. All support groups should have a trained professional that leads or facilitates the discussions (someone with experience and credentials). For more information, see Chapter 13 or to locate a group in your area go to www.apdaparkinson.org.

Legal and financial advisors

Your PD may eventually affect your ability to make key decisions about finances and legal matters, about the future of your family, and about your own future. Although this problem may never arise, working with an expert as early as possible after your diagnosis to put key documents and plans in order is just smart planning—whether you have PD or not. (For a full discussion of the legal and financial matters that need attention, see Chapter 20.)

Given the complexities of PD costs, drafting an insurance advisor for your team is a wise maneuver. This person can guide you and your care partner through the multitude of questions related to disability (short and long term), Medicare, Medicaid, Health Management Organizations (HMOs), Preferred Physician Organizations (PPOs), Health Savings Accounts (HSAs), and any other alphabet-soup plans that will undoubtedly surface in the future.

Spiritual advisor

Taking a holistic approach—caring for yourself physically, mentally, and spiritually—can give you a jump on managing your PD symptoms. Many people focus on the physical and mental but figure the spiritual will take care of itself. Remember: Your spiritual well being has just as many levels as your physical and mental health. If you have a spiritual mentor that you can tap to join your professional care team, do so early on. This person may be your clergy, someone who's mentored you through other passages, a practitioner of alternative or complementary medicine, or even the counselor that's mentioned in the "Psychologist or counselor" section of this chapter.

Making the cut

Drafting a team of experts in your battle against PD has benefits well beyond the expertise of each member. When you choose them carefully and treat them with respect, you find these men and women will go to great lengths for you. They even become some of your most enthusiastic cheerleaders, offering support and encouragement, humor, and affection as you confront the challenges of living with PD.

How do you evaluate each member of the team? The criteria are pretty standard—regardless of the profession:

- Does this person have the right stuff—the appropriate credentials and experience—to handle the job?

- Is it a good fit—are you comfortable with this person? Can you talk about anything or ask the silliest question without feeling intimidated?

- Does this person really listen? Is he open to ideas that aren't his own?

- Does this person give you the time you need—especially when your PD may slow your movements, thinking, and ability to put thoughts into words?

- Is this person willing to admit limits to her knowledge and expertise and refer you to someone more qualified to handle a specific issue?

- Will this person be there when you need him?

Working with Your Team to Manage the Unexpected

Stuff happens, and worst-case scenarios happen unexpectedly. Maybe you fall or burn yourself while preparing dinner and end up in the emergency room. Or, despite all precautions, you experience an adverse drug interaction that requires a stay in the hospital. Nonmedical emergencies—a fire, a weather event (such as a severe storm or tornado)—can also crop up. Our advice throughout this book is this: Have a plan in the event something unexpected happens. This doesn't mean you're assuming the worst. You just want to be ready—or as ready as possible.

Establishing an emergency plan

Be prepared—the motto of the Boy Scouts of America is just as useful for PWP and their care partners. You or your care partner may never need to dial 911, but what if...? Why not think in the relative calm of your normal routine and prepare for that possible unexpected event? These next sections provide specific recommendations to help you prepare and then deal with a variety of emergencies.

The home front
Start your emergency plan with home safety by reviewing the tips for accident-proofing your home in

Chapter 21. Then consider what to do in case of a medical emergency, such as an allergic reaction or a dislocated shoulder or some other emergency beyond your control—a fire, a flood, a blackout. Who do you call? Where do you go? What do you do?

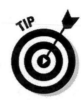

Your home is unique, just like you, so the best way to prepare for a safety emergency is to contact your local fire department. It may have a program where a firefighter comes out, assesses your home for fire safety, and then offers pointers for handling emergencies. Another resource that offers a checklist for creating your own evacuation plan is available through the American Red Cross at www.redcross.org.

Personal records

Take advantage of the following tips that put you ahead of the panic if a medical or safety emergency does arise:

- Gather this vital information:

- A list of all prescription and OTC medications and a list of any allergies and chronic health conditions you have besides your PD

- Insurance or Medicare numbers

- Your medical history

- Names and contact numbers of your doctors and for an emergency contact person, like your significant other, for example

• Date all this information and update it regularly, especially when you add or discontinue meds.

• Make sure you and your care partner have copies of this info at all times in your wallet or purse and in you car(s).

• Let key others (your employer, a trusted neighbor who may respond to an emergency) know where to find the information should you be unable to direct them.

> • Prepare a folder specifically for the emergency room. (People administering care don't have time to read old records.) Include the following pieces of information in the folder:

- All information listed in the previous section, "Personal records."

- A copy of your *advance directive* (a living will and a medical power of attorney), even if the hospital and your doctor already have it on file. If you don't want the medical staff to provide certain interventions or extraordinary measures to save your life, you must provide that information. (See Chapter 20 for more info on these and other legal issues.)

• Prepare a fireproof box with copies of key documents: insurance and Social Security cards; bank and credit card account numbers; wills, powers of attorney (financial and medical), and photos of valuables in case of a fire or weather catastrophe (such as a tornado or hurricane).

• Post critical emergency contact numbers near your home phone. Those numbers include local hospital emergency room, fire department, police department, utility company (for power outages), doctors, pharmacist (in the event of an adverse drug reaction), and a relative or friend to contact.

Easy access

You may never need emergency intervention, but you're better off to be prepared with information that an emergency team can readily access. Take the following measures to prevent glitches when seconds count.

- Distribute duplicate house keys to trusted friends and neighbors.

- Be sure your care partner can access financial funds any time you may not be able to take financial actions such as writing checks to pay bills or transferring funds from savings to checking accounts as needed.

- If you live alone, get a medical alert system, which enables you to call for help if you're unable to get to a telephone. (Yup, we're talking about that classic TV commercial—"Help! I've fallen and can't get up!")

164

Decision time

In an emergency, don't waste time worrying whether you should call for help. Risking a little embarrassment rather than your life is always the wise move.

However, if you do need to call for an ambulance or go to the emergency room, be realistic about your expectations. Keep in mind that the United States has nearly 40 million people with no health insurance; for these folks, the ER doctor is likely their doctor of choice.

Note: The Centers for Disease Control estimates the average waiting time in the ER (if you're not critically injured or ill) is three hours; in cold and flu season the wait can be much longer.

Because of possible delays, you need to

- Speak up if you're experiencing symptoms such as extreme pain, trouble breathing, dizziness, and other signs of distress.

- Tell every ER person who examines or assists you that you have PD (and any other chronic conditions such as diabetes or hypertension) even though someone has taken your history and you know these facts are on your patient information sheet.

- Be proactive. Make sure that the people who treat you are aware of your medications and allergies.

If your situation is serious but not life threatening, call your doctor or the nearest urgent-care or walk-in clinic for faster response and care. And if your doctor does advise you to get to the ER, he can speed up your process by calling the hospital and telling the ER staff that you're on the way.

The hospital stay and its aftermath

If you need to be admitted to the hospital, the cause isn't likely to be your PD. The more likely reasons will be a serious injury (such as a hip fracture or head trauma from a fall) or another heath condition (such as heart problems or diabetes). Regardless, be prepared with the necessary information (see the previous section for suggestions) to make the stay less stressful for everyone.

Leave valuables (checkbook, credit cards, jewelry, and the like) at home. If you must bring them because of an emergency and the haste in leaving for the hospital, hand them off to a trusted family member or friend as soon as possible. Or ask a staff member whether the hospital has a safe place to keep the valuables until you can make arrangements for them.

The same suggestions outlined for an emergency (see the previous section "Establishing an emergency plan") apply for a hospital stay. But, because you'll likely be in the hospital for days rather than hours, you must monitor the orders for your PD medications. The attending physician and the staff may not realize the importance of your PD meds' strict dosing and timing. For example, your neurologist's orders for medication at 8 a.m., noon, 4 p.m., and 8 p.m. may be interpreted by the hospital staff as four times a day over a 24hour period, or 8 a.m., 2 p.m., 8 p.m., and 2 a.m.

I'm not fooling around and I'm not drunk—I have Parkinson's disease

To offset any misunderstandings that may occur during your hospital stay, consider packing a copy of the following note in your bag and showing it to the staff. In spite of its lighthearted tone, the note provides critical information about your care.

To whom it may concern:

First of all, let me say how much I appreciate everything you'll be doing to care for me while I'm here. My care partner and I understand that you have other patients to attend to besides me. In return I ask that you understand some things about me:

• You may have noticed that I'm moving pretty slowly and I probably couldn't walk a straight line if my life depended on it. Am I intoxicated? Nope. I've got this thing called Parkinson's disease.

• Other times you may notice that I seem to be doing just fine—doing normal stuff like brushing my teeth, washing my face, walking around on my own—and then my call bell will light up, and I'll be asking you to please come help me get to the bathroom. What gives? I have Parkinson's, and the medications I take to control it have these *on-off* cycles. One minute I can perform routine things, and the next I need all the help I can get.

• Speaking of meds, I really need for you—and everyone involved in treating me while I'm here—to know that certain medications commonly used in hospital settings can really mess with my PD symptoms. Please check with my neurologist, Dr. _____ at _____, before ordering or administering any new medication—especially antinausea or antipsychotic meds.

• And finally, as long as the subject of antipsychotic is on the table, please be aware that my Parkinson's may cause me to experience confusion, disorientation, and even some interesting misperceptions about where I am and what you're doing. I may also start to hallucinate—fortunately these *visions* I experience are usually benign and silent, so no voices are suggesting that I do you bodily harm. Again please check with Dr. _____ before administering any meds.

That's pretty much it in a nutshell. Having PD and being in the hospital can be a challenge for both of us, but hopefully now that you understand, we'll both have an easier time of it. Thanks for understanding and thanks for your care and con-cern.

Sincerely,

(Put your name here)

Sometimes your PD meds need to be suspended so new medications for the condition that landed you in the hospital can work. Again, be vigilant about your care. Have your care partner alert your neurologist (or the doctor managing your PD care) as soon as you know you're going to the hospital and insist that the hospital on-call physician (or any doctor who orders the suspension of your PD meds) consults with your neurologist before ordering any changes in medication.

Any time that your medications are being administered *for* you (as in a hospital setting) instead of you taking them yourself, be sure that you or your care partner carefully examine the pills you get. If any of the meds look different from those you take at home, question it. Also, since hospital staff is responsible for administering medications to a number of patients with diverse conditions, there may be a delay in your getting your PD meds on time. If necessary, have your neurologist contact the attending physician at the hospital to discuss the correct medication regimen. Also, make sure the attending staff knows which medications may be *contraindicated* (harmful) for PWP. (Copy the list of red-flag medications provided on the Cheat Sheet at the front of this book and ask the admitting doctor to add it to your file.)

In addition to monitoring your medications, you may have another battle to wage: The hospital staff, even though they're medical professionals, may have limited or no experience with PD and may misinterpret your PD symptoms—on-off cycles, dykinesias, confusion from the stress of a hospital environment, and the like. For example, if a nursing assistant sees you up and mobile at 2:00 and comes back at 3:00 because you want assistance getting to the bathroom, he may think you're just looking for extra attention. For one good idea for heading off any staff resentment or misunderstanding, see the nearby sidebar, "I'm not fooling around and I'm not drunk—I have Parkinson's disease."

More tips for managing the unexpected

Emergencies arise for all kinds of people. But because you have PD, such crises may carry the extra elements of stress and panic. You and your care partner may want to consider taking a basic first-aid course through your local Red Cross or YMCA to better prepare yourselves for unlikely emergencies, such as bleeding, choking, medication reaction, falls, and so on.

If you need to call 911, be prepared to give the following information:

- Phone number you're calling from

- Address and directions to help the ambulance get there quickly

- Description of the person's condition (breathing? conscious?)

- Your name

In addition, follow these steps:

1. Don't hang up until the emergency operator tells you to.

2. Be sure you unlock the door and turn on outside lights.

Even if it's not night, the lit porch light makes locating the right house easier.

3. If possible, have another family member or neighbor wait outside to direct the emergency personnel.

4. Stay close so you can provide answers to key questions, but let the emergency personnel do their jobs.

5. Gather the information you've prepared (see the earlier section "Establishing an emergency plan") and get ready to go.

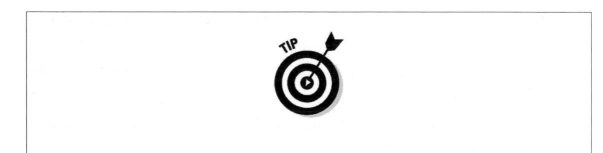

> Consider having only cordless phones so you can move around the house (unlocking doors and turning on lights) while you're talking on the phone with the doctor or emergency operator.

A Word for the PD Care Partner

This book has a number of chapters that you may want to read and heed. This is one of them. Putting together a network of professionals that you and the PWP can call upon as issues crop up will make life easier for both of you.

Within this group of professionals, you need to find your own experts—three people you can turn to with your concerns of managing and coping:

- **Primary care physician:** You may have the same general practitioner or internist as the PWP. As long as this physician attends to *your* needs and concerns when you're the patient, that's fine. However, you may want to consider a PCP who isn't involved in your PWP's care. This is your decision, but remember: You need someone to focus on maintaining your physical health and well being.

- **Counselor or therapist:** Being a partner in care can be extremely stressful, especially as the needs escalate. But you'll be better prepared to cope with the unexpected twists and turns along the way if you take time now to connect with a professional who counsels care partners. Don't be stubborn about this. You are at risk for episodes of anxiety, panic, and depression as much as the PWP.

- **Support group and spiritual advisor:** Okay, so we cheated and lumped two into one. But your spiritual health is a vital piece of your ability to partner in care. A support group can provide a safe place to talk about (and let go of) those bad feelings you may be wrestling with (see Chapter 22 for more on this topic). And it has folks who can laugh and share some of the black humor that comes with being a care partner—they all know, understand, and feel your pain. As for a spiritual advisor, you know yourself best. Your clergyperson, a trusted mentor, your counselor or therapist, and your support-group leader are all good candidates to fill this role.

Chapter 7

Choosing How and When to Share Your News

In This Chapter

• Setting a course with your care partner

• Keeping the story straight: How to share the news with your family

• Sharing with your inner circle: That's what friends are for

• Determining who else needs to know

• Taking the high road: People who overreact and folks who poke their noses in your business

---

Living with Parkinson's disease (PD) can go well beyond the person diagnosed with PD. Day in and year out, the disease also affects the people who live with, work with, care about, and love the person with PD (PWP). It affects generations—children, grandchildren, and even aging parents (in the case of young onset PD, see Chapter 8), who may be facing their own health challenges.

Everyone has concentric circles of personal contacts. In the closest circles, we have our immediate family (spouse, partner, kids, parents) and perhaps a couple of truly best friends. Next comes a little wider circle—friends we socialize with, extended family, and perhaps a couple of professionals, like our doctor or clergyperson. Further removed from the core of our lives is another group—our employer and co-workers, acquaintances, and neighbors. Deciding when and how to tell each person or group about your diagnosis is an individual decision, one that you have to base on the dynamics of your relationships and your comfort level in sharing this kind of news. But first...

Before You Start Spreading the News

Even if you initially share your diagnosis with very few people, you need to plan how you want these people to react—both immediately and in the future.

Establishing your ground rules

Start by determining your ground rules and the level of support you want. The following categories identify some of the more common PWP stances:

- Some PWP are fighters: They go on immediate offense, take charge, and fight this enemy with every ounce of strength and all the resources they can muster.

- Other PWP take a flight (or more defensive) position: In some ways they choose to ignore the whole situation. Flight folks use their energy and resources to assure everyone (and most of all themselves) that nothing has really changed—life goes on.

- A third group of PWP falls somewhere in the middle, combining facets of fight and flight: Although they want life to continue as normally as possible, they realize they have to fight back to keep their PD's progression at bay.

Whichever group you're in, you need to think about your ground rules for living with PD. What kind of meaningful care and support can the groups of people in your life offer as you face life with PD? Those who care about you—family members, friends, neighbors, co-workers—naturally want to help. In many cases, they're not sure how to offer that support. You need to explain the ground rules and indicate what will—and won't—be helpful.

Preparing to state your needs

Think through now—alone, or preferably with your care partner (the person who will most likely be with you for the whole journey)—how other people can help. Initially you may need people to listen, to distract you when necessary, and to give you the gift of normalcy just by being themselves.

As your needs become more specific and as you accept the hands-on help of others, you also discover three really important outcomes:

- You empower people by allowing them to contribute something truly meaningful to you.

- You ease some of the responsibility that may have fallen on your care partner's shoulders.

- You prevent yourself from becoming isolated, and you actually increase your ability to take control of situations as they arise.

Accepting help is not a sign of weakness; in fact, it's a sign of strength. Acceptance shows you haven't surrendered to the challenges of PD. And when you can't fight the battle alone, you still win because you have people willing to step up to the fight for you.

Meeting the challenge with good humor

We can't say this too often: An upbeat, optimistic attitude is one of your most effective weapons against PD. And right next to it is the ability to laugh—with others, at yourself, and especially at your PD. We're talking black humor here, folks.

Bill of Rights for people with Parkinson's

Declarations of individual rights are nothing new. Perhaps you've noticed *rights* lists posted when you visit a hospital or care facility. But we think it's important that you—the person with PD—know your own inalienable rights. Feel free to edit and add your own ideas to the following list. Then bookmark it and reread it regularly.

I have the right

180

- To take care of and make decisions for myself for as long as I am capable and to expect my care partners to respect my wishes, should the time come when they speak for me

- To seek help from others as I recognize limits to my own endurance and strength

- To maintain those facets of my life that were part of my identity before my PD diagnosis for as long as possible—even if each task takes three times as long

- To occasionally (and humanly) get angry, be depressed, and work my way through other difficult feelings

- To reject any attempt by others (either consciously or unconsciously) to limit my independence because it'll make life easier for them

- To expect and receive consideration, respect, encouragement, affection, and forgiveness as long as I offer these same qualities in return

- To take joy and pride in my accomplishments—regardless of how small—and the courage it takes to achieve them

> • To speak out and demand that new resources and eventually a cure be found—if not for me, then for those who follow

For example, a diet-center leader famous for her wonderful sense of humor inspired her feeling-sorry-for-themselves clients with the story of her father, a large, barrel-chested man who had always been bigger than life. Then he got cancer and started fading away—literally. One day toward the very end, when he was but a shadow of his former robust self, he said to his daughter, "You know I want to be cremated." She nodded in agreement. "Well," he added, "if I keep dwindling away like this, I think you'll be able to do the job in the microwave!" His daughter was first stunned and then burst into laughter. That's black humor, folks – and it works because it helps you keep your perspective as you face the sometimes tough days of living with PD.

Breaking the News to Your Care Partner

Chances are your care partner was with you when the diagnosis of PD was confirmed. If you learned the news together, then the telling part is done. But the two of you still need to spend some time working your way through the questions of how this diagnosis is going to affect your lives—individually and together.

If your primary care partner is not your significant other (perhaps she's a sibling or an adult child who works, has a family of her own, and lives in another community), give yourself a day or so to digest the diagnosis and think about how you prefer to break the news.

When you're ready (don't wait too long; a day or week at most), try to have the conversation in person and allow enough time to work through the discussion. If you can't talk in person, choose a time when this person isn't distracted by other activities and have the discussion by phone. When you deliver the news, reassure this person that the diagnosis is not life-threatening and you have no need for immediate action. Then set a time when the two of you can discuss your present needs, your needs down the road, and her willingness and capability for fulfilling those needs.

If you have to deliver the initial news by phone, urge your care partner to check out some of the Web sites in Appendix B. Or call the folks at the National Parkinson Foundation at 800-327-4545

and ask them to send copies of their excellent (and free) booklet, *Parkinson's Disease: Caring and Coping* to both of you. (In fact, while you're at it, ask for copies of the entire series of booklets.)

During this sit-down conversation with your care partner, allow enough time to:

- Share immediate emotional reactions—even if you've had a couple of days or a week since you and your care partner heard the news.

- Be prepared for different responses. One of you may react with denial and the other with anger. (Before this discussion, you may both benefit by reading the section on personality differences in Chapter 5.)

- Set down in writing a list of steps to take. Include a tentative timeline for each one based on the tips we offer in the next section.

Resist the urge (by you or your care partner) to leap ahead and take dramatic and life-changing actions such as putting your home up for sale and moving in with your daughter or assuming that you need to quit your job. You have time. You are years—and perhaps decades—from needing to make these lifestyle changes because of your PD.

Telling Your Family

When and how you deliver the news to your immediate and extended family is an individual choice that's influenced by

- The status of individual family relationships.

- Your personal feelings about how soon you want even close relatives to know.

When you're ready to talk to family members, the easiest way may be a family gathering (if geography allows) where you tell all the adult members at once. Everyone can hear the same version, and details won't get distorted through repetition. However, because families are so spread out in today's world, a family meeting may not be possible. In that case, consider arranging a conference call. Again, the goal is to deliver the news to all the adults at the same time.

If you have children, find a place and time to share your news with them before that larger meeting, especially if your PD is of the young-onset variety and your children are still living at home. Your children will make this journey with you; they deserve to have the same time and privacy to digest this news as your care partner had.

Give adults the facts

When you deliver the news to the adults in your immediate and extended family, stick to the basics:

- What PD is

- Whether others in the family are at risk

- How PD is treated

- What your prognosis is

Some family members may have suspected a serious illness of some kind; others may be completely shocked at the news and take it hard. In either case, a good first step is to educate and inform.

PD associations offer a number of basic educational and informational materials for fundamental questions about PD. These excellent materials are listed in Appendix B. Handing out this printed information at a family meeting (or e-mailing it if your family lives elsewhere) gives them a reference for questions after the initial shock wears off. By selecting the same material for everyone, you lessen the chances of that information becoming distorted.

Set a positive tone

After you share the facts of PD with adult family members, consider setting the tone for your emerging new relationships. For example, you can add, "There's a lot I don't know, but I do know I can live a relatively normal life in spite of my symptoms. The tough part is figuring out how to live it without people feeling sorry for me or treating me differently." With that simple statement you've laid out the ground rules:

- You have PD, but you're still you.

- Most important, you want other people to continue treating you the same. (Okay, so Cousin Fred can let you win a few more poker games and your mother may finally call someone else to get the cat out of the tree each week.)

- How much you say beyond that—symptoms, research, no present cures and such—is strictly up to you and your assessment of how much information this group can handle at the first telling.

When that question of "What can I do to help?" comes up, perhaps the best answer is to make these three points:

- Help me by being yourself and finding ways to continue our relationship as normally and fully as before.

- Help me make sure my care partner maintains a life outside of mine.

- Help me most of all by understanding that I'm still the same person inside. Don't let my PD symptoms scare you or make you treat me any differently.

Don't sugarcoat the situation for kids

Today's children are bombarded with information from every possible angle. Put another way, this generation is far savvier at a far younger age than most adults can imagine. On some level, even very young children can understand that something has changed in their environment. Don't underestimate their capacity for feeling stress and tension, especially when they can sense the undercurrent in the household but no one's talking with them about it.

• Teenagers can usually handle the same information you give the adults. If your teen is especially sensitive or perhaps struggling with other emotional challenges (the break-up of a relationship or not making the sports team, for example), you may want to have the conversation with that teen separately so you can focus on reassuring and comforting her.

• With younger children (or grandchildren), keep details as simple as possible. A terrific resource for telling young children (under age 12) about PD is the book entitled *I'll Hold Your Hand So You Won't Fall: A Child's Guide to Parkinson's Disease* by Rasheda Ali and her father, Muhammad Ali.

• In some cases, children in their middle years (ages 9 to 12) are mature enough to be included with the adults in the general family meeting. But just because they seem to understand and accept the news, don't assume that they don't have concerns or a gazillion questions about how your lives are going to change.

- If the child is your grandchild, decide with the parents the best way to deliver the news.

Regardless of the ages (or seeming maturity) of the children, never forget that they're children; they haven't lived long enough to pile up the life experiences and tools for coping that an adult has. Check in with your children and grandchildren often through positive techniques such as:

- Seeking their help with innovative ways you can cope with certain limits to normal tasks (like dressing) when your PD symptoms hinder you

- Continuing to pursue activities the two of you have always enjoyed—even if you have to find ways to adapt, such as getting a recumbent bicycle instead of riding your old one

- Providing the opportunity (place and time) for them to raise questions and concerns about what your PD means for the future

Giving Close Friends the News

Soon after you break the news to your family, consider how and when to tell your closest friends. Again several issues are at play here, including the fact that friends may have already noticed your symptoms and discussed their concerns with each other. They may not have brought their concern to you directly because they didn't want to intrude.

How and when you choose to tell this group depends in part on the nature of the group. In other words if your close friends are also close with each other, then inviting everyone over to your house and telling them all at the same time may be best. The advantage is that everyone hears the same words (although they may process them differently) at the same time directly from you. In addition, they can see your response to the diagnosis—hopefully upbeat and optimistic—at the same time. And they can all hear the ground rules for how you want them to respond to your diagnosis.

In cases where you have close friends who are not close with each other or friends who live in other places, you may want to tell each individually. If so, try to do it face to face (or at least by phone—not e-mail) so the person can see and hear how you're handling the diagnosis.

Consider providing the same helpful information (fact sheet and list of Web sites) that we identify in the two previous sections so your friends can pursue questions that may occur after you tell them.

Friendships can be critical to your overall sense of control and well-being when you're living with PD. Unfortunately, a lot of PWP make the mistake when they get the diagnosis of pulling away from their friends or denying their need for that support (tangible support like cutting the lawn or intangible support like just being there to listen).

When PWPs (or their care partners) react as if the support is an insult or a statement of the PWP's incapacity, they make matters worse. This reaction can have a snowball effect because the friend who wanted to help feels rejected (even embarrassed) at apparently adding to your stress. Before you know it, those treasured friendships (along with the normalcy and pleasure they brought your life) have disappeared.

As soon as you and your care partner are ready to go public with your news to friends, take control and set the tone by doing the following:

- State your needs regarding your approach to PD. For example, tell them you understand that they may want to rush in and start helping you (preparing meals, handling the household and yard chores, and such), but the best support they can offer is to help you maintain as normal a life (and relationship) as possible for as long as possible.

- Appreciate any offer of support and help (even if you shudder to think that they believe you need that help).

- Be prepared to suggest alternate ways they can be a part of your network of support and caring.

Another way to think of outside help is to consider your care partner and his soon-to-be-filled-to-capacity schedule. By maintaining a normal routine with friends and associates, you give your care partner a break to pursue life aside from PD.

When you respond to your friends' invitations to activities you enjoyed before PD with "I can't...," they may stop offering and gradually get on with their own lives. Instead, try an attitude of "I'd love to [play cards, bike, meet you at the coffeehouse]. Help me figure out how we can make that happen." Then you can brainstorm options together.

As Lance Armstrong (the seven-time Tour de France winner and cancer survivor) has said, "C'mon, man. *Everything's* an option."

Widening the Circle: Informing Others

On the outer fringes of those concentric circles we describe at the beginning of this chapter are those people who play a role in your life but not a vital or intimate one (neighbors, community group associates, professionals you rely upon, and so on). Breaking the news to this last circle of contacts (with the possible exception of your boss and co-workers; see Chapter 16 for the specifics on that special group) is not a responsibility that you need to feel compelled to do right away—or ever. Basically, your condition's really none of their business.

On the other hand, don't underestimate the unexpected support and management resources that may come from one of these people. For example, your barber or beautician may offer to make a house call as your symptoms change. Or your neighbor may be happy to be on call for emergencies when you're alone and your partner's at work.

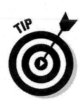

When the timing seems right during the first months following your diagnosis, let these people know you have PD. Only you can decide how much information they need or what kind of support and response they may provide. But, as with anyone you tell, be prepared to set the tone for their response, to correct misinformation they may have about PD, and to appreciate their concern and support however they express it.

Handling Sticky Conversations

Having said that, we need to get real here. Some people (and they may be in your closest circles) are more hindrance than help when they hear you have PD. One type simply can't handle bad news of any sort, so you end up spending a lot of time and energy comforting and emotionally supporting their (mostly unfounded) fears and anxieties. Another type believes they have all the answers even though they have zero real knowledge about PD. They, too, can use up your resources of energy and good humor as you try and educate them to the realities of living with PD. Consider these tips for handling those sticky situations:

• For people who simply can't cope with difficult news, consider being prepared with a specific request. You can ask, for example, "You're such an avid biker, would you be willing to bike with me once a week? My doctor tells me that exercise, especially now in the early stages, is really important, but I'd rather not go out alone."

If this person is a close friend or family member, you may want to speak with him separately and acknowledge his obvious fears and anxieties. Then let him know that he can be most helpful by trying to remain upbeat and positive—at least in your presence.

If all else fails, allow such people an initial period of mourning over your news. Then insist that they get over it or else you'll have to limit your contact with them. This is not about these people. You're the one with PD and, bluntly stated, you just don't need other people bringing you down.

• For the well-meaning folks (even strangers!) who see your tremor or some other PD symptom and start telling you the story of their uncle's wife's brother who also had PD, you need a different tactic. No doubt such people mean well, but they'll never be part of your care team. This empathy and advice (or showing off!) is about them, not you.

Don't allow unwanted advice or comments to upset you. Of the two of you, *you* are the expert at PD. Acknowledge their effort to help, and then walk away.

Chapter 8

Special Advice for Those with Young Onset Parkinson's Disease

---

In This Chapter

• Noting similarities and differences of YOPD and traditional PD

• Fleshing out problems unique to YOPD

• Incorporating financial security into the plan

• Refining the PD care partner's role

When it comes to Parkinson's disease (PD), no one's more famous than the popular actor Michael J. Fox. The twinkle in his eye and his legendary self-deprecating humor—even about life with PD—make him less the celebrity and more the national support-group leader for millions of people with Parkinson's (PWP) and their care partners.

In a 2006 interview in *AARP, The Magazine,* Fox reported that as many as 40 percent of the 60,000 new PD cases each year involve someone younger than age 50. This figure alone blows holes in the myth that only old people get PD. The fact that Fox was first diagnosed in his 30s shines an even brighter light on the growing numbers of young and active people who face this challenge.

The cause of *young onset Parkinson's disease (YOPD)* is as debatable as the cause of traditional onset PD (see Chapter 2). But what isn't debatable is the fact that it hits people in their prime, plays havoc with their established roles (spouse, parent, adult child of aging parents), derails rising careers, and over-rides plans for the future.

In this chapter we take a look at the specific issues facing people diagnosed with YOPD. When the information is the same for any PWP, we refer you to other chapters in the book. But if you're 30, 40, 50, or not yet 60 and have PD, this chapter's for you.

Comparing YOPD to Traditional Onset PD

The term *onset age* means when symptoms first appear—not when a diagnosis is made. If the onset age is earlier than age 50, the diagnosis is usually YOPD. (In very rare cases, PD symptoms appear before a person reaches the age of 21; the term *juvenile Parkinson's* distinguishes it from traditional or YOPD.)

Two excellent resources for information specially aimed at people with YOPD are Young Onset Parkinson's Association (YOPA) at www.yopa.org and The Michael J. Fox Foundation at www.michael jfox.org, where you can sign up to receive regular *Fox Flash* e-mail bulletins. These periodic updates cover upcoming foundation activities and provide valuable tips and information for PWP and their care partners.

How they're the same

PD is chronic, progressive, and (at least at this writing) incurable regardless of your age and when you get it. On the positive side, it's possible to live for many years—in some cases a regular lifespan—in spite of having PD. It's possible to continue to work, to raise a family, to see children marry and have children of their own, and to enjoy many of the same activities you enjoyed before being diagnosed.

How they differ

YOPD and traditional onset PD differ in three basic ways:

• People with YOPD are less likely to experience the dementia (memory problems) or balance problems that affect people whose PD begins when they're older. Part of the reason for the difference is that older people are more likely to have multiple conditions (such as Alzheimer's, a series of small strokes, or adverse medication interaction) that affect memory and balance.

• People with YOPD may experience a condition known as *dystonia* (unusual muscle cramping, aches, or abnormal movement in a particular area of the body such as a foot or shoulder). For reasons that still aren't clear, older patients seldom experience dystonia but tend to have *tremor* (shaking), a symptom that's less common for a person with YOPD.

Although dystonia is well recognized as the possible first symptom of YOPD, your diagnosis may be delayed if your doctor isn't familiar with such PD symptoms in younger patients. According to the Young Onset Parkinson's Association, the number of people with YOPD may be significantly under-reported for the very reason that many people experience early symptoms for years before they get to a doctor who considers PD as a possible diagnosis.

• In general, people with YOPD appear to respond well to antiparkinsonian medications, yet side effects (such as *dyskinesia*—uncontrollable movements) may affect them more quickly than older PWP.

In an article for the American Parkinson's Disease Association, Lawrence I. Golbe notes that people with YOPD experience two specific medication-related problems more than older PWP: early wearing-off of the medication benefits and on-off fluctuations (when PD meds lose their effectiveness so symptoms reappear before the next dose is due).

Many people with YOPD (and their doctors) elect to postpone treatment with antiparkinsonian meds as long as possible to avoid some of these escalated symptoms and side effects. **Note:** Research shows no clear evidence that early withholding of therapy has long-term benefits.

Faster or slower? What's the prognosis?

The jury's still out on the pace of progression for people with YOPD. However, more advanced therapies may eventually postpone the progression of symptoms

202

for a longer time—perhaps adding years to the person's relatively normal life.

PD—regardless of the age of onset—affects each individual differently. As with any health issue, your physical and mental health at the onset of PD (and your fight to maintain that well being through a balanced diet and regular exercise program) can have an enormous effect on the prognosis. Nothing is carved in stone regarding the progression of symptoms—no matter how old or young you are when they start.

Facing the Special Challenges of YOPD

If you have YOPD, the most difficult challenge may be the very fact that you're young. You had planned a life packed with many goals, and one of them was *not* living with a chronic and progressive condition!

Most people in their young adult years tend to see themselves as invincible. They may take steps to ensure financial security for their family and themselves in the unlikely event that something bad happens, but they really don't consider it a possibility.

But, now it appears that the *unlikely* event has happened: You've been diagnosed with YOPD. And it's standing directly in the way of the life you've planned. At first you can see no way around it. But you know better. You know something this scary, this bleak can enrich your life in many ways.

Stop for a moment and consider other times when you faced what seemed like an impossible challenge. How did you respond to that challenge? Maybe it was a basketball game when your team was down by a point with only seconds to go and you were at the line for two free throws. Maybe it was a far more serious situation like financial difficulties or the possibility of losing your job. Maybe it was when you needed and wanted to prove yourself to someone you admired and respected. Whatever the challenge, you took some mental steps early on to face the threat or achieve what you wanted.

In this section we give you the mental steps to help you get through this diagnosis and come out on top—again.

Getting an accurate diagnosis

The diagnosis of YOPD is based on the same cardinal signs used to diagnose PD at any age:

- Tremor at rest (trembling when body part is not engaged in activity)

- Rigidity (muscle and joint stiffness)

- Bradykinesia (slowed or impaired ability to move)

- Postural instability (impaired balance)

Cases of YOPD tend to present less often with tremor and more often with bradykinesia, rigidity, and abnormal muscle cramps (dystonia) that frequently affect one foot.

When a person develops PD at a young age, the doctor must make sure that the patient doesn't have another disorder that can mimic parkinsonism (see also Chapter 4). Your doctor should always check for two rare diseases in particular: *Wilson's disease* (which requires a different treatment) and *Dopa-responsive dystonia* (DRD), which has a prognosis very different from PD.

The genetic element (see Chapter 2) seems to be more prevalent in YOPD than older PD patients. In some cases, the doctor may order a test for *Parkin* mutation, which is more frequent in YOPD. If you agree to have this DNA test, be sure you ask to see a certified genetic consultant in order to discuss all the implications (emotional and practical) of this test for you and your family.

Handling the diagnosis: A positive attitude is the best offense

Get ready for a ride on the emotional roller coaster after you get the diagnosis. Your initial reaction may range from disbelief to denial to anger to all of the above and then some. Your mind may rocket from image to image—will you see your kids grow up, graduate, and marry? Will you be able to work and support yourself and your family? What about the dreams you had of traveling, starting your own business, running that marathon? What about those words *no cure?*

Give yourself some time to mourn the fact that your life does not—for the moment—seem to be headed in the direction you had hoped. And then get on with it. This is the life you've been given. Everyone has to deal with challenges and tough choices at some point in life. PD is yours.

Because you're under 50 (even under 40), you have young onset PD, which has no cure—yet. However,

• Researchers have already developed proven techniques and therapies for managing and treating symptoms.

• You can maintain function and a relatively normal lifestyle over a period of years and—in your case—possibly decades.

• You will not die from Parkinson's disease

• Much of the life you imagined is still within your reach. The odds are very good that you'll

- See your children grow up, graduate, marry—and have children.

- Continue working for years to come and even realize the dream of starting a second career.

- Travel. Why not? (The marathon may be a little trickier.)

- Get very good at finding ways to adapt PD to goals that are really important to you.

And the best defense is a good offense

Okay, so you've taken time to digest the diagnosis and you have the attitude thing going. Now what? Take a look at the following sections to keep moving in the right direction.

Brain power

You initial response may be to run to the library or computer and look at every statistic you can find on YOPD. What were the odds that you'd get PD? What's the likely prognosis in years? What percentage of PWP your age are able to keep working, see their children grow up, have sex?

Mark Twain said there are three kinds of lies—lies, damned lies, and statistics. You can choose to believe the statistics and project them onto the rest of your life or you can refuse to be a statistic. You can determine that you're unique and that you'll custom design (with your care team—see Chapter 6) your PD management for you—and only you. But the immediate challenge is to get to work educating yourself (and your family and friends) about this diagnosis.

You've already taken a positive step by reading this book! It's chock-full of chapters offering information for anyone living with PD—young or not-so-young. After you've read it (and, of course, shared it with people close to you!), keep it handy. As you make this journey with PD, use this book as a guide to the resources you'll need along the way.

Carpe diem: Seize the day!
The overriding emotion you may feel early on is a sense that you've totally lost control of your life. But you can only lose control if you surrender to it—if you choose to hand it over to someone else and simply follow other people's orders. There's a better approach to PD for you and your care partner—one that gives you the best chance of living the life you planned before the diagnosis.

Take charge of this thing—the same way you'd attack any other unlikely event (like losing your job or your home being damaged by fire). Life can hand you bigger problems than PD—really! Unlike people facing a terminal illness, you have time and a reminder to be proactive and do what matters most now, not some day.

Without going all the way to Pollyanna-mode, consider the advantages of a can-do and optimistic outlook:

- The very fact that time becomes more precious can instill the determination not to waste an hour or a day.

- Close relationships can be strengthened—marriages, parent-child connections (yours as a parent and yours as the child of aging parents).

- Genuine and dedicated friends will stick; hangers-on will not (and you may be surprised at who's who in the bunch).

- New people—interesting and stimulating, understanding and fun—come into your life.

- There's nothing like a progressive illness to make you get off your butt, take that trip, write that novel, or go back to school.

- You now have the opportunity to work with other people to make a real difference in the lives of millions. How many people do you know who can say that?

- In some ways you're getting a fresh start—the chance to change you. Suddenly you understand in a very real way that life *is* finite.

Staying on track in your career

A question that's bound to be at the top of your mind is whether or not you can continue working. On so many levels, your ability to pursue a career, run a business, or maintain financial security is integral to living the life you envisioned. Be sure to read Chapter 16 for a full discussion of PD in the workplace.

One of the key messages you want to send to your employer, co-workers, and yourself is that the prognosis of YOPD is good. With proper management of PD symptoms through exercise, diet, and medications, your career can be good to go for years to come. When your neurologist, physical therapist, and nutritionist fully understand your job's requirements, they can structure your care plan (and timing of meds when you begin taking them) to provide optimal function when you need it most.

Before you sit down with your employer to discuss your diagnosis and its possible effects on your work, plan ahead by

- Exploring options such as flexible hours or telecommuting. If your employer makes such options available to other employees (like new parents or regular part-timers), then you're not asking for special consideration.

- Thinking through the demands of your specific job and how to handle them. Anticipate the questions (and doubts) your employer may have about your ability to continue.

If you think it's necessary, ask your neurologist to prepare a letter that explains the status of your PD in relation to your work.

Stress can pack a double whammy when it comes to maintaining your job and career because stress comes with the territory in many (make that *most*) jobs and can do a real number on your YOPD symptoms. Take a look at Chapter 16 for ways to manage stressful situations in the workplace—this is a huge step toward successfully maintaining your position for years to come.

Dealing with PD's impact on relationships

Now that you have PD, your diagnosis can become the two-ton gorilla in the room, sitting squarely between you and other people—if you let it. When you fear that your lover, child, best friend, or co-worker can't see you because PD's in the way, then take the initiative. Make sure these people remember that you're still you! By addressing PD issues that may affect your most important relationships, you can remove that gorilla from the room.

Your role as a spouse or significant other
The roles you and your partner have settled into may undergo quite a make-over as your PD progresses. Fortunately, this progression usually occurs over a period of years with ample time to adjust. But that delay doesn't mean you can't or shouldn't prepare for

necessary changes. In other words, begin communicating now. Communication and patience are your best resources for adapting later to these inevitable changes. These are some examples:

- If your tremor worsens and you've been chief handyperson for the household, how's that going to work out? Talk about ways that you can manage the task with more time, or use this opportunity to teach a child how to wield a hammer.

- If small, cramped handwriting is an early symptom of your PD and you're the lead check writer and bookkeeper, can that continue indefinitely? Maybe you can pay bills online or install software to print out checks that you only need to sign.

- If you've been the family's gourmet cook but now you take hours longer to turn out one of your signature meals, then you (and those around you) need to practice patience by allowing for the extra time you need. Then again, you may consider graciously (and willingly) accepting some help.

> Don't rush into changes before they're necessary. Do take time to plan with your partner the ways that you can adjust certain tasks or roles before you give them up.

As your symptoms progress and your medication timing switches unexpectedly into on-off mode, your spouse or significant other may find it tough to believe you're suddenly struggling with a task that you managed fine just a minute earlier. Be honest about what's going on. Acknowledge that it looks like you don't want to do this task, but—for now—you really can't. Communication and patience are paramount here!

Another common concern when you have YOPD is the question of intimacy. Okay, to put it bluntly—you're wondering about its impact on your ability to perform sexually. The answer: If you experience a change in your sexual desire, performance, or pleasure, a host of underlying causes are possible. Some of the more common ones are:

- Side effects of medications

- Effects of certain cardiovascular conditions (high blood pressure, circulatory problems, reduced blood flow, heart disease and such)

- Impact of other conditions such as urinary incontinence, menopause for women, or prostate problems for men

- Effects of depression, stress, or anxiety

- Symptoms common to PD (tremor, stiffness, on-off episodes, dyskinesias and such) that can affect movement (not to mention the mood!)

PD may cause sexual dysfunction, but this symptom usually occurs several years into the progression of the disease, and other symptoms (including those listed above) can play a role. Don't simply assume that a change in your desire for intimacy or ability to make love is a normal part of PD. Solutions are available, so talk to your doctor and look at Chapter 19 for more information on sexual dysfunction.

Intimacy means more than the act of making love. Think about the progression of your relationship. Maybe it began with flirting and progressed to the sheer romance of the courtship before you two

216

decided you were in this for the long haul. Maybe you surprised your partner with an unexpected romantic gesture—flowers for no reason, holding hands at the movies, the funny card, or handwritten note. Rekindle those little moments that led to falling in love and the commitment of a long-term (or even lifetime) relationship.

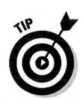

Maintain a sense of humor. Surely even at your healthiest you had those moments—embarrassing, silly, laugh-out-loud times when it all went hay-wire at a critical moment. Plan to roll with them. Shared laughter can be incredibly sexy.

Your role as a parent

How life may change for you and your kids will depend on their ages when you're diagnosed. If they're very young, you can keep the news simple and guide your children as they grow up and your symptoms progress.

By the time they reach their middle or high school years, living with a parent who has PD will seem so normal that it'll be their friends' parents who seem different.

If your children are older (middle or high school) when you're diagnosed, communication may be more difficult. At this age your children are dealing with a lot already. They're trying to locate their own sense of identity among their peers and within the family unit, they're trying to live up to adult expectations, and they're facing ever-escalating pressure to make the right choices. No wonder they shut down sometimes!

Now you come along and deliver the news that you have PD—a disease they may have heard about but one that they may have some real misinformation on. Depending on their age and your relationship, your children may or may not ask questions, but don't assume that they have none. On the other hand, dole out information carefully. You may hear "TMI!" (too much information) from your teen when you start throwing around terms like *bradykinesia, substantia nigra,* and such.

If you have teens or middle-schoolers, you may want to ask for help in researching information. They're undoubtedly proficient on the computer. Give them a focused PD topic to research and ask them to share it with the family. For example, put them to work locating and bookmarking the best PD Web sites for the family. What organizations can they find? What are the strengths of each site? By proactively including your children in a management plan for your PD, you take away a lot of their fear and distress that can come from being left out of key discussions and decisions.

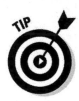

Your role as a friend

If you're fortunate enough to have a network of close friends—even if that network is only two or three people—you have a fabulous resource for coping with your PD. Friends can listen when you really don't want to burden your spouse or significant other. And they can take your focus off PD to get you back on the track of living the life you'd planned. Friends can make you laugh and let you cry. They can push, shove, and irritate you until you'll do anything to get them off your case. They can admire your courage, wonder at your ability to contain this beast, and celebrate each passage—just as they did when you didn't have PD, and just as you've done for them.

Friendship is a two-way street. Your friends can only be there if you let them, and they'll be there for the long term only if you let them know you'll do the same for them. For more ideas on PD and friendships, see Chapter 15.

Your role as a co-worker/employee/employer

By some estimates, up to one-third of PWP (at any age) are actively employed. As the news of your diagnosis spreads at work, your co-workers will probably take one of two positions: Some will immediately come forward, express their concern, and ask what they can do to help; others will pull back, take a let's-see-how-this-goes position.

As with all your relationships, this one is yours to manage. Frankly, your best bet is to let people know that you have PD (after you've told your employer). Otherwise the rumor mill is going to be the messenger. Consider sitting down with members of your department (with your supervisor's approval) to give them some brief, basic facts about YOPD. You can then ask these co-workers to use these facts to squelch rumors they may be hearing.

If you're the employer (or department head), be aware of immediate employee concerns for you *and* for themselves. What does your PD mean for the future of the business and their job security? Again carefully prepare by anticipating questions and concerns (from good employees seeking other positions or ambitious staffers eyeing your position) for you and your business.

Whatever your job, you need to realistically assess (and reassess regularly and frequently) your ability to handle the job. Your greatest barrier will be stress, and the greatest stress comes when people around you clearly question your ability to do the job. For ways you can address this problem and the related challenges of PD in the workplace, see Chapter 16.

Your role in the community

Over time your PD becomes more and more difficult to disguise. Even if you can manage the outward symptoms like a tremor or impaired movement, the stress of trying to keep it a secret can drain you. But why expend so much energy to keep people in the dark when they may become unexpected sources for support and outright help?

Maintaining (or instigating) community relationships isn't just about the personal returns. When you volunteer at your child's school or join in for a charity walk or bike event, you're making a better world for others—and that's empowering. You're not this poor PWP; you're someone who chooses to take advantage of an opportunity to make a real difference for yourself and the community around you.

Speaking of community action, the Parkinson community—national, regional and local—is well organized and a great place to get involved. By taking an active role in advocating for more research dollars, better therapies, and eventually a cure, you empower yourself and other PWP. Not a marcher or the outspoken sort? Not a problem. Check out www .parkinsonaction.org or any of the national organizations listed in the appendix of this book for ways you can get involved behind the scenes.

The Dollars and Cents of YOPD Financial Planning

Definition of *terrifying:* The experience of a person in the prime of life getting news that he has a chronic and progressively debilitating illness. Although people with YOPD can hope for a cure in their lifetime, basing their financial futures on such a pipedream is, unfortunately, unrealistic.

Realistically you'll live with PD for many years to come, years that may include getting married, raising a family, sending kids off to college, securing the future for your partner, caring for aging parents—a host of emotional and financial challenges. Our suggestion? Regardless of your economic status, take your partner and get to a financial planner now (see Chapter 21 for tips on choosing one) to help you plan for the future.

If you're in debt now, you need a plan to manage that debt and end it as quickly as possible. If you have plans for major financial commitments (such as buying a car or home or sending your child to college), you need to ask yourself whether such plans are still viable.

Financial planning is one of those tasks where preparing for the worst scenario is the wisest move. You may ask, "But what if I never need to put the plans in action?" The best answer is a different, more challenging question: What if you *do* need to?

If you haven't already done so, take time to ask the big questions:

- What are my current health insurance plan's benefits?

- What hospitalization, disability benefits, and programs may be available through my work?

- What are the benefits and limitations of the COBRA program if I have to stop working?

- What long-term care insurance program can I (or my partner) benefit from?

- Am I eligible for that program?

Connecting with other YOPDers

"I have plenty of friends," you say, "so I don't need to connect." Oh, but you do. You have a condition that usually strikes people decades older than you. You have a chronic, progressive condition that's going to impact every facet of your life. On top of that, you have this life—of work and relationships and social events and community functions and.... So, you're going to have times over the coming months and years when the very person you need to talk with is someone who understands what it means to have YOPD, someone who's been there, who's still there—someone who can tell you to knock it off, stop wasting precious time, and get on with your life when you start feeling sorry for yourself.

So where can you find these people? If you're really fortunate, a YOPD support group is close enough for you to conveniently attend meetings. If it isn't, then check with the facilitator of any PD support group that meets in your area to see how many of the participants have YOPD. If that fails, ask your neurologist whether she treats other YOPD patients. If she does, perhaps names and contact information can be exchanged.

Your best resource may be the Internet. One established organization specifically for YOPDers is Movers and Shakers at www.pdadvocates.org The Parkinson Action Network at www.parkinsonsaction.org is another great place to connect with PWP of all ages. The National Parkinson Foundation at www.parkins on.org sponsors an annual conference for YOPDers and their families. In addition, chat rooms and other sites offer people with YOPD a chance to connect—even in the wee hours of the morning. Two such sites are www.braintalk.org and www.plwp.or g.

The point is that you (and your care partner) can connect with others your age that understand and have experienced or are experiencing many of the same frustrations you are. Your friends and family members may be terrific—supportive and concerned—but how can they possibly understand the full impact of YOPD? Not even your neurologist can fully appreciate what it means to have PD in the prime of your life.

Connecting with YOPDers isn't about giving up on friendships that have sustained you (and that still sustain you). But connecting with other YOPDers can lessen your sense of isolation and provide you with resources and news to manage your symptoms in a variety of situations. Another person with YOPD may not become your new best friend—but then again, don't rule out the possibility.

226

If you have no insurance, talk to your financial planner immediately about options that may be available in your state or through federal programs. If the financial planner can't answer your questions or provide information in a timely manner, find another planner!

In addition to your financial planning, take the following measures to help your medical providers:

- Establish a *durable* power of attorney for healthcare decisions as well as financial decisions.

- Write a living will or advance directive; make sure you distribute copies to every doctor who treats you and carry a copy with you in case you need to go to the hospital or emergency room.

- Be sure that the people you appoint to speak for you know what you want them to say and do!

For a more detailed discussion of legal and financial concerns that need your attention sooner rather than later, turn to Chapter 20.

A Word for the PD Care Partner

When you discover that someone you love has a condition that takes that person's functions and abilities, your instinct may be to go into full caregiver-mode and take charge. Please resist that urge! The person you love is exactly the same person that he was before the diagnosis. PD doesn't change a person overnight. In fact, the changes are gradual enough for the two of you to take the time to adapt, prepare, and plan.

But you don't want to run away either. Throughout this book we talk about the fight-or-flight response to tough situations. If you're a person who takes flight (backs away and finds reasons to become disengaged), then you need to reassess that instinct. The person you love and are devoted to needs you—your support and understanding—in the early going, and she may eventually need more of you as her spokesperson and advocate.

If you're a fighter (a person who takes charge or refuses to lose), you may need to dial it down a notch or two. Although you're the care partner, the operative word is *partner.* You're not in charge; you don't have YOPD. Contribute and discuss options—yes. Coax and encourage—absolutely. Defend your right to a life beyond your partner's PD—positively. But in the final analysis, the person with PD has the right (as well as the ability) to decide how she wants to face this challenge. It's called *patient autonomy* and it's the very foundation of medical ethics.

Part III

Crafting a Treatment Plan Just for You

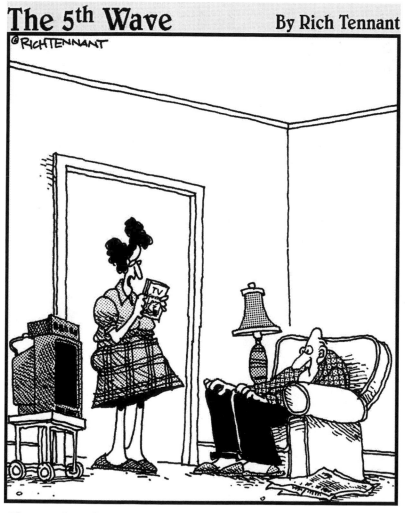

"Well Dad, if you're feeling down why don't you watch some TV. Let's see, there's 'Silent Killers', 'When Puppies Attack', and 'War of the Worlds.'"

In this part...

You can explore the variety of options available to treat your PD and help manage symptoms. These include medications and surgery as well as complementary and alternative medical treatments. Our chapter on diet and exercise includes an illustrated program of stretching and strengthening exercises that you can take to your doctor or physical therapist for review. Finally we have a chapter on clinical trials where we discuss the pros and cons of participating in such projects and what you need to know before you make a commitment.

Chapter 9

Managing PD Symptoms with Prescription Medicines

In This Chapter

• Grasping the lowdown on meds for PD's motor symptoms

• Minimizing those non-motor symptoms

• Getting (and staying!) squared away on your meds

Your Parkinson's disease (PD) diagnosis will include treatment options for managing your symptoms. If you have no symptoms of functional disability at the time of your diagnosis (in other words, if the PD isn't interfering with your ability to live your normal life), then your doctor will most likely prescribe programs like exercise and nutrition counseling, a support group, and, of course, regular visits to his office to monitor symptoms and any signs of progression.

As your symptoms begin to affect your work, social, and routine activities, your doctor will likely add *pharmacologic* therapy (prescription medications) to the treatment plan. In this chapter, we look at the most common medications for managing symptoms, some that have been around for decades and others that are relatively new to the scene. We also pass along some suggestions for staying on top of your medication regimen.

Because PD has no cure at this time and there is no means of preventing its progression, the treatment goal is to manage the symptoms, postpone their progression, and minimize the onset of new symptoms for as long as possible.

Managing Motor Symptoms with Proven Prescription Medication

In managing your symptoms, your doctor may prescribe a variety of medications to help prolong your current level of function. The medication may be available only as a brand-name drug (meaning it's still under patent protection), or it may be available in the generic form (meaning the patent has expired). Brand drugs are usually newer, more expensive, and possibly more beneficial than generics.

All medications for PD have one goal: to restore brain concentration of dopamine to near-normal levels. To achieve this goal, your doctor may prescribe one or more pills with different mechanisms of action (similar to different foods that we routinely use to restore sugar levels in our body, such as pasta, fruit, and sweets). The number of pills doesn't necessarily correlate to the gravity of the disease!

Almost 40 years after its introduction, the combination of *levodopa* and *carbidopa* (usually prescribed under the brand name *Sinemet*) is still the preferred treatment for most people with Parkinson's (PWP). The following sections cover the components of this medication and the role each one plays.

L-dopa—The gold standard

The most effective prescription medication to date for controlling PD symptoms is *levodopa* (often abbreviated to *L-dopa*), which brain cells use to produce more *dopamine,* the neurotransmitter that PD reduces. Producing more dopamine permits relief for PD symptoms such as stiffness, tremor (shaking), facial mask, cramped handwriting, slow movement, and impaired gait (walking).

Historically, L-dopa was administered alone, which caused a whole list of side effects including nausea, loss of appetite, vomiting, lowered blood pressure (leading to dizziness and possible falls), and rapid heart rate. Because these side effects were so significant, researchers almost dropped L-dopa from the regimen before they discovered the advantages of prescribing it with its now-conventional partner, *carbidopa.* Coupled with carbidopa, L-dopa can almost completely control PD symptoms for a *honeymoon* period of two to eight years.

Unfortunately, 50 percent of PWP develop motor complications after 5 years of levodopa therapy; virtually all of them experience a decline in the benefit of levodopa after 10 to 15 years of therapy.

Carbidopa—L-dopa's companion

Any time the treatment seems worse than the condition, researchers look for ways to make the treatment more palatable for the patient. Carbidopa's main purpose is to offset the serious and uncomfortable side effects of levodopa without causing side effects of its own. In addition, carbidopa

- Allows your system to absorb the essential vitamin B6

- Lessens the amount of levodopa you need to control symptoms

When your symptoms do require medication, the prescription will probably be a low dose of carbidopa/levodopa. The prescription includes two numbers—usually 25/100. The first number refers to the amount of carbidopa and the second is the amount of levodopa. Your doctor monitors your symptoms on this low dose (usually taken at regular intervals three to four times a day). If you experience side effects, he can double the amount of carbidopa in your prescription. As the symptoms of PD progress, your doctor may increase the dosage and shorten the periods between doses.

Two other formulations for this medication are:

- The controlled-release (CR) form of Sinemet, which prolongs the effect of levodopa

- The orally disintegrating tablet (ODT) form of carbidopa/levodopa(brand name *Parcopa*)

With ODT delivery systems, you place the tablet on your tongue and it melts (like a mint) in a matter of seconds without water.

Entacapone—Another bodyguard for L-dopa

Recently a new class of drugs, *catechol-O-methyl transferase* inhibitors (COMT-I), has been added to PD therapy. COMT-I blocks the enzyme 3-O-methyldopa and allows even more levodopa to reach the brain. (Imagine levodopa with two body guards—carbidopa and *entacapone* or *tolcapone* (see the following paragraph)—to shelter it from dangerous enzymes on its journey toward the brain.) Other advantages of adding COMT-I to L-dopa are

- Longer duration of the L-dopa effectiveness

- Potential for reducing the dosage of carbidopa/levodopa

- The possibility of managing *off* times more effectively (See "Tracking the on-off fluctuations of your meds" later in this chapter.)

Entacapone (brand name *Stalevo*) is a new L-dopa therapy that combines the COMPT-I with carbidopa/levodopa. This three-in-one combination makes dosing easier because you take one pill, not two. Another COMT-I, *tolcapone* (brand name *Tasmar*), is available but has some limitations associated with liver toxicity.

Other effective prescription medicines

Your doctor may prescribe other medications in addition to your carbidopa/levodopa to better manage your symptoms. We cover the most common classes of these companion drugs in the following sections.

Dopamine agonists (DA)

Unlike levodopa, which is transformed into dopamine, *dopamine agonists (DA)* imitate the characteristics of dopamine. Your doctor may recommend that you try a DA before prescribing Sinemet as a first-line treatment in order to delay the complications associated with the use of levodopa over the long haul. (See the previous section "L-dopa—the gold standard" for more about Sinemet.) DAs have been in use for two decades with proven effectiveness in treating PD symptoms. But their use may be limited by troubling side effects, such as daytime sleepiness, low blood pressure, edema (swollen feet), vivid dreams, and, on occasion, hallucinations.

Four dopamine agonists are available. Older generation drugs (bromocriptine and pergolide) are rarely used because of possible cardiac side effects. But newer generations of DAs (including *pramipexole* and *ropinirole*) offer effective management of symptoms with relatively fewer side effects.

Of the four DA medications available, studies haven't proven one to be more effective than another. Therefore, if you have an unfavorable response to one DA, ask your doctor about trying a different one to see whether it's more successful.

Monoamine oxidase inhibitors (MAOI)

This class of drugs works by interacting with monoamines, chemicals in the brain that transmit messages between nerve cells. Of the three monoamines (dopamine, serotonin, and norepinephrine), dopamine is the focus for PWP because it controls messages related to movement.

Although MAOI has two subtypes (Type A and Type B), only MAOI-B is used to treat PD. Its fundamental task is to inhibit the *oxidation* (burning) of dopamine, which clears the dopamine from the *synaptic space* (the tiny space between brain cells where chemical messages are exchanged). As a consequence, more dopamine is available and PD symptoms improve. Interestingly, MAOI-B may provide an additional benefit by acting as a kind of neuroprotector (see Chapter 2), possibly slowing the progression of PD and delaying the need for carbidopa/levodopa therapy.

The original drug from this group is *selegiline,* which doctors still prescribe for the early stages of PD because it provides some control of PD symptoms. A new formula of orally disintegrating selegiline *(Zelapar)* has recently been introduced with a lower incidence of side effects and a once-a-day dosing schedule. The most recent drug in this class to receive FDA approval is *rasagiline* (brand name *Azilect*), also taken once a day for the treatment of early PD. For PWP in the moderate to advanced stages, a combination of selegiline and L-dopa can improve symptoms.

The downside to MAOIs is their potentially serious effect on blood pressure, especially when the patient is taking other medicines that also affect blood pressure. Take these precautions to avoid serious problems:

- Be sure all doctors know you're on this medication and always check with your pharmacist before using:

  • Over-the-counter (OTC) products such as cold-cough remedies (especially those including *dextromethorphan*) and diet supplements

  • Prescription medicines such as antidepressants that increase serotonin levels

- If you're scheduled for surgery, be sure the anesthesiologist knows you're taking rasagiline because anesthesia combined with the MAOIs can cause a dangerous drop in blood pressure.

- Be aware that MAOIs can cause abnormalities of blood pressure known as *tyramine* (or cheese *effect*) when the patient is eating aged cheese or drinking red wine.

Consult your doctor if you have additional questions about the serious side effects of MAOIs.

Transdermal patch—A new delivery system

In most cases, prescribed medications come in a tablet or capsule form. But researchers are working on other ways to get the drug into your system with improved effectiveness, fewer side effects, and a shorter waiting period before the drug takes effect.

As one example of such research, at this writing the Food and Drug Administration (FDA) is in the process of reviewing a *transdermal* (skin) patch for the delivery of rotigotine, a dopamine agonist. You apply the patch to your skin (back, shoulder, or abdomen) once a day. The advantage of the patch is its consistent delivery of medication throughout the day. Consistent delivery of the dopamine agonist helps smooth out the amount of medicine you receive unlike the peaks and valleys that occur when taking tablets or capsules multiple times each day. This new method may improve symptom control and reduce side effects. Patches for the delivery of levodopa are also under study.

Amantadine

Amantadine is another older medication that doctors occasionally prescribe in early stages of PD because it can provide some benefit before levodopa is needed. Exactly how amantadine helps relieve symptoms isn't clear. In fact, it was originally (and continues to be) a treatment for the flu, but scientists serendipitously stumbled on its potential PD benefits. Most recently doctors have noted amantadine's benefits in managing *dyskinesia* (the writhing, twisting of the body) that may occur after long-term levodopa therapy.

Keeping the names straight

Your doctor has a growing arsenal of medications with which to treat your PD symptoms. Table 9-1 provides a handy reference for their generic and brand names.

Table 9-1: Generic and Brand Names of Common PD medications

Class of Drug	Generic Name	Brand Name
Carbidopa/Levodopa		
	Carbidopa/levodopa	Sinemet
	Carbidopa/levodopa controlled-release	Sinemet CR
	Carbidopa/levodopa/entacapone	Stalevo
	Carbidopa/levodopa orally disintegrating tablet (ODT)	Parcopa
Dopamine Agonists (DA)		
	Bromocriptine	Parlodel
	Pergolide	Permax
	Pramipexole	Mirapex
	Ropinirole	Requip
	Rotigotine (transdermal system)	Neupro
COMT Inhibitors		
	Entacapone	Comtan
	Tolcapone	Tasmar
MAO-B Inhibitors		
	Selegiline	Eldepryl
	Selegiline ODT	Zelapar
	Rasagiline	Azilect
Others	Amantadine	Symmetrel

Treating Non-Motor PD Symptoms

PWP must deal with a whole range of symptoms—only some of which involve movement. In the chapters that follow, we discuss in detail the PD symptoms of depression and anxiety and symptoms that may occur as your PD progresses. (See Chapters 13 and 19.) However, if any of the following non-motor symptoms become disruptive to your routine and life, talk to your doctor about medications that may be helpful:

• **Dizziness or changes in blood pressure when you stand after lying down or sitting:** Report this to your doctor! Treatment may include changes in habits (such as increasing fluid intake or wearing support stockings) or a change in medications.

• **Increased saliva or swallowing problems:** Again, your doctor needs to know about this because it may be a side effect of a medication or it may be the progression of your PD. Either way, don't ignore it!

- **Sleep disturbances:** The disease itself and some of your antiparkinsonian meds can cause sleep disturbance. Ask your doctor whether a sleep aid may be helpful. In some cases where sleep disturbances are especially troublesome, a more specific sleep study may be indicated.

- **Pain, cramping, or dyskinesia:** These symptoms are often worse at night or bedtime. A change in your evening dose of Sinemet (higher or lower) may solve the problem, or ask your doctor whether anti-inflammatories (such as ibuprofen), muscle relaxants, or dopamine agonists may help.

- **Nausea, stomach upset, constipation, and heartburn:** These symptoms may be part and parcel of your medication routine. Talk to your doctor about when, how often, and to what degree of discomfort these symptoms occur.

- **Urinary frequency or urgency:** Conditions other than your PD (such as prostate hypertrophy) may be at play here. Talk to your doctor if you experience any change in urinary habits, especially if you experience pain or any sort of discharge with urinating.

If you're seeing another doctor or taking medication for high blood pressure or another chronic condition, be sure your neurologist and all doctors consult with each other before prescribing new meds for you.

Using Your Medication Safely and Effectively

As a person with PD, you need to pay close attention to your medication timing and dosing. You also need to be aware of changes in performance and function (mental or physical), especially if such changes seem to relate to your medication routine. In short, you need to

- Take an active role in monitoring your medications and the results you get (or don't get) from them.

- Inform your doctor and pharmacist of any side effects, new symptoms, or worsening of current symptoms.

This section covers the important ways you can work with your doctors and pharmacist to maintain a healthy regimen with your meds. We also pass along some advice for keeping track of your meds and their effectiveness with your PD symptoms.

Partnering with your doctor and pharmacist

Work with your neurologist to review *all* your medications from time to time. Be sure to include any OTC products you take regularly. And remember to pay special attention to any dosing changes or new prescription meds another doctor may have ordered.

When your neurologist and other doctors write a new prescription for you, ask the following questions:

- Why are you prescribing this medication at this time?

- What results should I expect after I begin taking this medication?

- How soon should I expect positive results?

- How should I take the medication—timing, dosing, with (or without) food and so on?

- What side effects might I experience?

Keeping the costs of meds under control

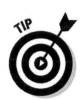

If the cost of your medications is overwhelming, you may be eligible to receive some of your prescription medications for a reduced cost or even for free. The American Parkinson Disease Association (APDA) partners with a coalition of health providers, pharmaceutical companies, patient advocacy groups, and other organizations to help you get the medicine you need. Call 888-477-2669 or go online to www.pparx.org for full details on eligibility. You can also check with your state Office on Aging or go to www.benefitscheckup.org or www.needymed s.com for more information.

• What side effects should I notify my doctor about immediately?

• What side effects would require me to get to an emergency room or call 911?

• What does the medication cost?

• Can I get the same benefits a less expensive way?

For example, Stalevo is convenient but can be expensive. Taking Sinemet and Comtan separately may save money.

• Are any interactions possible between the new medication and other prescription or OTC meds that I'm already taking?

When you get the medication the first time, be sure the pharmacist prints out and reviews the prescribing information sheet with you. (If you don't have a regular pharmacist, ask your neurologist to recommend pharmacies in your area that she respects and communicates well with.)

Before you leave the pharmacy:

• **Ask questions if anything on the information sheet raises a red flag for you.** For example, if a side effect of the new med is low blood pressure and you're taking medication to manage high blood pressure, how will the new drug affect it?

• **Check the label to be sure you can read it and that you have received the right medication according to your doctor's instructions.** If a substitution has been made (a generic for the brand your doctor prescribed, for example), ask the pharmacist to call the doctor to be sure the switch is okay.

• **Open the package and look at the medicine, especially if it's a refill.** If the pill or tablet doesn't look like the med you've been taking, immediately bring that question to your pharmacist's attention.

Mixing prescription and OTC medications

Pick up any magazine these days and you'll likely find an article touting the advantages of some herbal supplement or vitamin. Or maybe a friend recommends some OTC product for your heartburn, headache, or cold symptoms. The question is: How will these commonly used products interact with your prescription meds—especially your antiparkinsonian meds?

Anyone who takes a prescription medication to manage or treat a chronic illness needs to vigilantly read labels on all OTC as well as prescription products for potential interactions. Call the primary care physician or neurologist and talk to the pharmacist before taking the meds to let these professionals help you decide if this med is right for you.

Common signs of potentially dangerous drug interaction include accelerated or slower heart rate, diarrhea or constipation, heartburn, nausea or cramping, fever, skin rashes or unusual bruising, dizziness, confusion, loss of appetite, or abnormal fatigue. If you experience any such side effects, contact your doctor. If side effects are severe—or a doctor is unavailable—call 911 or get to an emergency room.

Note: Ask your doctor whether grapefruit juice can have an effect on your medications. Studies have shown that grapefruit juice can interfere with the liver's ability to break down some medicines—especially prescription drugs.

Balancing the benefits of medications against their potential side effects is delicate. In partnership with your doctor, determine what combination works best for your lifestyle and quality of life. The goal is to keep you *in* control—as opposed to *under* the control—of your meds and your PD.

Setting up a routine for managing your meds

Being human, we have a tendency to ignore or bend the rules, especially when it comes to faithfully following a medication regimen. We skip doses, miss the timing by a couple of hours, cut the dose to save money, and even share prescription meds with other people (because it did so much good for us).

With PD, taking medicine and taking it in the prescribed and timely manner is critical. And, because you probably take more than one medication for PD (not to mention the meds you may take for other conditions such as high blood pressure), timing is indeed everything.

As your PD progresses, you may experience memory problems, so it's enormously important that you figure out now how you're going to remember to take your meds. This section offers suggestions for both organizing your medication regimen and remembering it.

Three keys to avoid problems with your medications:

• Make sure one (and only one) doctor (your neurologist is the best choice) oversees all your medications, including OTC vitamins, supplements, or herbal remedies.

• Choose one pharmacy (or one pharmacy chain that maintains your records regardless of where you are) to fill all your prescriptions.

• Take a list—if not the actual meds—to every doctor's appointment (including dentists, podiatrists, and so on) and to the hospital or emergency room if you need to go there.

Hospitals use several medications to combat nausea following anesthetic that are *contraindicated* (or *not to be used*) for PWP. These drugs not only worsen PD symptoms but can actually produce Parkinson-like symptoms in people with no diagnosis of PD. For a complete list of these drugs, see the Cheat Sheet in front of the book.

You also need to get organized at home—where you most likely take your meds. You've probably seen or even used those plastic pill-containers that organize meds by day (or even by dose throughout the day). Some of these containers come with a beeper that signals the time for a dose. Other varieties have large sections to accommodate several pills or larger pills.

Consult with your pharmacist on the best choice in medication organizers for your purposes. Think about your daily activities:

• Are you home all the time?

If you are, then one large, multi-sectioned container may be a good choice.

• Are you at work when one dose comes due?

Then a smaller pocket container or one with the reminder alarm is a good choice for that dose.

Establish a regular time (the same time and day every week) for loading the meds into the proper container. Then place the container(s) in the most obvious place to remind you. (For example, you may want your morning and bed-time meds next to your toothbrush.)

Tracking the on-off fluctuations of your meds

As if multiple motor, cognitive, and other symptoms of PD aren't enough, the common PD medications can also affect the course of the disease. Read any PD article or get into a discussion with any PD patient or care partner, and sooner or later you hear the terms *wearing off* and *on-off.*

The *wearing-off* effect may appear when the PWP has been on the same dosage for some time. Over time, the positive effect of the med simply wears off before the next dose. In that window between the end-of-dose benefit and the delivery of the next dose, the PWP may experience heightened symptoms of PD, such as tremors, difficulties with balance and coordination, and so on. Such incidents commonly occur after a relatively long *honeymoon,* when the antiparkinsonian meds effectively control the symptoms. The usual solution is to shorten the time between doses, increase the dose, and/or add other meds.

The *on-off* phenomenon (which is fairly unique to PD) refers to the PWP's ability to perform common physical activities one minute and then be totally incapable the next minute, all within the same dosing cycle. Another way of looking at this phenomenon is that the wearing off effect loses its predictability so

PD symptoms emerge without warning. Some PWP actually refer to the sensation as someone flipping a switch. Usually this effect occurs when the PD is in the advanced stages.

We recommend that you track your on-off fluctuations after they begin by noting the following and reporting your findings to your doctor:

- The time the meds start wearing off in relation to your next scheduled dose of medicine.

- The exact symptoms that reappear.

- The frequency of the off-period. Is it every dose or just now and then? If it's now and then, is there a recurring pattern?

Finally, *dyskinesia* (involuntary movements) is another treatment-related symptom that may become apparent as the disease progresses. Movements may range from dance-like to irregular and jerky motions, and they usually occur when the medication dose is at its height.

For friends and family, this seemingly random ability of the PWP to act normal one minute and need help the next minute may appear calculated, to gather sympathy or manipulate other people. But the cause is simply not known. Recent theories link the continued loss of dopamine-producing cells and years of drug therapy as a possible cause. Both the PWP as well as family and friends must understand that this on-off effect isn't within the PWP's control, isn't a deliberate attempt to gain sympathy, and may not respond to a change in the medication routine.

Chapter 10

When Surgery Is an Option

In This Chapter

- Sizing up your chances for successful surgery

- Checking out the advances in surgical options

- Stepping through the deep brain stimulation process

- R & R: Life with your DBS

As Parkinson's disease (PD) progresses, medications often lose their effectiveness; sometimes they cause, rather than alleviate, problems for the patient. In these instances, surgery may bring much-needed relief and even restore some level of normalcy to the patient's functions and life for many years. In this chapter, we explore current surgical procedures and raise the important questions for you to ask before deciding to proceed.

Deciding Whether You're a Candidate for Surgery

First things first: Of the many people with Parkinson's (PWP), which ones are more likely candidates for surgery? The following questions are a general guide to help you understand your chances for a successful outcome from surgery.

- Have you successfully used antiparkinsonian medications (primarily L-dopa therapy) for several years?

- In spite of an optimal medication regimen, are you experiencing increasing freezing episodes (sudden difficulty in moving), on-off fluctuations (shortened time between response to meds and time for next dose), and dyskinesia (twisting motion—a major side effect of taking the antiparkinsonian meds)?

- Is your tremor so severe that medication can't control it?

Of course, your age, past medical history, and general health are always considerations before deciding to undergo surgery, but you're more likely to benefit from surgery if you answered "Yes" to all of the above questions.

Note: Unfortunately, PWP whose main issues involve cognitive loss, impaired balance that doesn't respond to L-dopa, poor speech *(dysarthria),* or swallowing problems *(dysphagia)* are less likely to be helped by surgery.

Even if you appear to be a prime candidate, you have a great deal to consider before deciding whether surgery's right for you. Most importantly, remember that you may experience relief—even significant relief—of some symptoms, but your PD will progress. In particular, symptoms that surgery can't address (such as autonomic dysfunction or cognitive decline) may still be a factor in the progression of your PD.

On the other hand, if certain symptoms (like tremor, bradykinesia, dyskinesia, rigidity, and on-off fluctuations) have begun to rule your life, surgery may buy you some much-needed relief and time to enjoy a higher quality of life. This isn't a decision you or your doctor should make lightly.

Weighing Your Surgical Options

At this writing, surgical options for treating PD are virtually limited to *deep brain stimulation* or DBS (see section below). But scientists continue to seek new procedures that may prove more effective in controlling symptoms or stopping them altogether, allowing the patient to remain symptom-free for a period of time. (See the sidebar "Stem Cell Research: The Controversy" later in this chapter.)

Deep brain stimulation (DBS)

The new standard for surgical treatment is a process called deep brain stimulation. Since the FDA approved DBS in 2002, over 25,000 PWP have had the procedure. In addition, DBS can effectively treat other neurological conditions such as essential tremor and dystonia (See Chapter 4 for more information.) Follow-up studies have shown consistent benefits for up to five years. However given the relatively recent introduction of DBS to PD therapy, the long-term safety and effectiveness of this procedure is still being studied.

According to a 2004 report from the University of Florida Movement Disorders Center, of 174

PWP referred to the center as candidates for DBS, only eight met the criteria that indicated they could benefit from the procedure. Proper screening by a medical team experienced in DBS is essential.

During the DBS procedure, a specially trained surgeon implants a *neurostimulator* (a battery-operated device similar to a pacemaker) to send electrical stimulation to those areas of the brain that control movement. The procedure follows these steps:

1. The surgeon drills a small hole in the skull and then inserts an electrode (called a lead), positioning it in a targeted area of the brain.

2. The surgeon then inserts an implantable neurostimulator (sometimes called a pulse generator or IPG), or battery pack, under the skin in the area of your collarbone.

3. In a procedure that takes place two to four weeks after the implant of the lead, a thin, in-

sulated wire (called the extension) connects the battery pack to the lead.

4. Your neurostimulator is then programmed to send signals appropriate to your individual condition and symptoms. (Several sessions may be necessary to get the programming right for you.)

Advantages of DBS include:

- The possibility to tune the device at any time in order to maximize benefits and minimize side effects

- A significant reduction in the amount of medication you need

- Significant relief from the troublesome side effects (such as dyskinesia) of those medicines

- The possibility of reversing the procedure in the future if a new, more promising procedure becomes available

Downsides of DBS include the following:

• This is still brain surgery with potentially severe—though rare when DBS experts perform the surgery—complications, including the potential for brain hemorrhage (bleeding).

• DBS isn't intended to stop the progression of your PD, although long-term studies are needed to clarify the long-term benefits of DBS.

• Two significant factors you must consider are cost and proximity to the center where the procedure is performed.

Find out in advance whether your insurance covers the cost of DBS. Also make plans for making the trips to and from the DBS center for follow-up visits.

Lesion procedures

Procedures such as *pallidotomy* and *thalamotomy* were the earliest surgical procedures to relieve PD symptoms.

• Pallidotomy destroys (or *lesions*) the *globus pallidus* (a part of the brain that becomes overactive in PD) in an effort to restore movement control.

- Thalamotomy is a similar surgery aimed at controlling tremor by surgically destroying a selected portion of the brain's thalamus.

Despite some encouraging results in the 1980s and 1990s, doctors recommend these lesion surgeries much less frequently today because benefits tend to regress after five years. In addition, serious side effects (such as difficulty in speaking, poor balance, and cognitive dysfunction) are possible, especially if the surgery is on both sides of the brain. Unlike DBS, these procedures are not reversible and will probably prevent the patient from taking advantage of more effective surgeries in the future.

However, for a small number of patients, this procedure may be more appropriate. Candidates include patients with poor access to programming and continued follow up after DBS, patients with higher risk of infections from a foreign body, and patients that—for one reason or another—can't have a stimulator.

Gamma knife surgery

Gamma knife surgery is an alternative technique for pallidotomies and thalamotomies in PWPs. Not a knife at all, the gamma knife is actually a machine that uses powerful, focused beams of radiation to precisely target the specific area of the brain. The procedure is usually on an outpatient basis, takes under an hour, and uses only local anesthetic. According to a study from Emory University in Atlanta, although lasting benefits in some patients have been reported, gamma knife surgery may have a higher complication rate than has previously been indicated due to delayed onset and under-reporting of changes.

Looking to the future: Surgical possibilities

Scientists are working on improvements to DBS, focusing on such details as a smaller and longer-lasting battery pack or a battery pack in the electrode so everything operates as one unit in the scalp. Another possibility is providing branch leads in the stimulator that network to various parts of the brain that control movements.

Stem cell research: The controversy

Until scientists can prevent the loss of or repair damage to dopamine-producing brain cells, PD will continue to be a chronic and progressive disease. This is where the controversial topic of stem cell research comes into play. Actor Christopher Reeve was an outspoken and tireless advocate for stem cell research, believing it was the only hope for people with brain or spinal injuries. Other spokespeople in favor of stem cell research include former first lady Nancy Reagan for Alzheimer's disease, Mary Tyler Moore for juvenile diabetes, and of course, Michael J. Fox for PD.

The debate is not only scientific but ethical. Scientists have ample evidence that cell transplantation may be the key to curing or preventively treating millions of people suffering from various conditions. In a nutshell, stem cell research focuses on transplanting renewable cells to replace lost or damaged cells due to problems such as chronic and progressive conditions, brain or spinal injuries, and the like. However, as researchers begin using human subjects to test the cell-transplant models already proven in animals, the need for a renewable supply of stem cells from human fetuses creates a heated debate.

Opponents' primary argument is that these cells are part of a viable fetus; therefore taking them is the same as aborting a human life. Further, they argue that scientists have no real evidence that cell transplants will work, especially in diseases like PD, where the root cause is unknown. People in favor of stem cell research argue that stem cell research isn't limited to finding cures; it focuses on the larger arena of understanding, preventing, and treating disease more effectively.

Scott Stern, associate professor of management and strategy at Northwestern University's Kellogg School of Management sums it up this way: "To stop stem cell research now because there are no immediate applications would be like stopping work on transistors in 1947 when their main application was considered as a potential hearing aid."

For more information on the stem cell debate, go to www.parkinsonaction.org or www.michaeljfox.org.

Beyond DBS, researchers hope to prevent, stop, or even reverse the death of dopamine-producing cells through advances in gene therapy and cell regeneration. (See the sidebar in this section, "Stem cell research: The controversy.")

Undergoing Deep Brain Stimulation

Brain surgery is pretty scary, but it certainly places a whole new light on managing PD's symptoms and living a full and functional life for as long as possible. Keep in mind that this surgery is elective—it's *your* call, not the doctor's.

Note: Because DBS has virtually replaced all previous types of surgeries to treat PD, we focus on it in the remaining pages of this chapter.

Asking the right questions before DBS

Regardless of what your doctor tells you, this decision is yours to make. So take time to educate yourself (and your family), and consider this surgery from all points of view.

Before making a decision, take advantage of the following suggestions:

- Read the literature your doctor offers, and educate yourself fully about the procedure, the benefits, and the risks. Get written information about possible complications and risks. A primary question to ask is, "Can DBS make my PD worse?"

- Meet with your neurologist and the neurosurgeon. As with any potential surgery, ask questions and expect definitive answers about the risks and worst case scenario. (For example, less than 5 percent of patients will experience serious complications, such as stroke or bleeding, from DBS surgery, but a slightly higher percentage may develop an infection at the implantation sites.)

- Ask the neurosurgeon what percentage of his total practice are DBS procedures. Also ask whether the surgeon has ever been sued for mal-practice related to a DBS procedure and how many procedures he has performed.

- Ask the neurosurgeon who will follow up with you after the implant. Does he collaborate with an experienced programmer and movement-disorder specialist to manage the settings on your neurostimulator? Is he part of an established DBS program or does he work on his own?

- Ask your neurologist (or your support-group facilitator) to introduce you to two other patients who have had the procedure—at least one of whom is a few years postsurgery. Talk to those patients about their experiences before, during, and after the surgery.

If you decide to go forward after weighing all the pros and cons of surgery, read on so you and your family know what to expect.

Passing the presurgical tests

Before your procedure can be scheduled, you need to pass several presurgical tests. These tests are fairly standardized and usually include a general medical examination to be sure you're healthy enough to endure the stresses of surgery; neuropsychological testing to be sure you don't have dementia and are emotionally and mentally prepared; brain imaging tests (such as an MRI or CT scan); and the usual blood tests, electrocardiogram, chest X-ray, and such.

Ironing out the details

After successful preliminary testing, the next step is scheduling the procedure. DBS is never an emergency, so the surgery date should be based on the surgeon's schedule and availability but also on your (and your family's) convenience.

Before the doctors get to work on your brain, cover the following two issues:

• Everyone involved in the surgery and postsurgical care needs to be aware of your medications (for PD and anything else). Be sure a clear plan is in place for managing all your medications (including those for other conditions, such as high blood pressure or diabetes) during post-surgical care and throughout your recovery.

See the Cheat Sheet inside the front cover for a list of common post-surgery drugs that can be a real problem for PWP in the postsurgical recovery period.

272

• Make sure your family knows when and where they can expect to see the doctor following surgery.

Knowing what to expect during and after surgery

Okay, everyone's in place and ready to go. The day of surgery isn't too pleasant, but then surgery's rarely a walk in the park.

For three to six hours, you'll be under local (or possibly no) anesthetic, off your medication, aware of your surroundings and the doctors, and experiencing the full range of your PD symptoms. The good news is that you'll be so integrally involved in the procedure—answering questions from the surgeon and other people as they work—that you'll probably be less aware of the discomfort than you imagine. (Prior to surgery, your doctor can provide printed information and a full description of the procedure).

Because DBS requires precise work, your head will be in a helmet-like contraption that attaches to your skull and the operating table to ensure that your head remains still throughout the procedure. (Sounds like something out of a sci-fi or horror movie, but in most cases, the only complaint is a post-surgery headache.)

The steps necessary to implant the neurostimulator are precise and demanding. Fortunately modern technology has special brain-imaging equipment that permits your surgeon to calculate the precise coordinates of the targeted area deep in the brain. In addition, most centers proceed to *map* your brain activity by recording the electrical activity of different groups of cells encountered during the journey from the surface to the depth of the brain. In fact, every area of the brain has a distinctive electrical *language,* which allows the surgeon to match the initial coordinates with the proper area activity. (Someone has compared this process to a tourist traveling blindfolded through Europe trying to identify his position based on the local language.)

After the lead is in place (see the previous section "Weighing Your Surgical Options" for more about this process), your surgeon may implant the battery and extension wire at the same time or wait up to a week before connecting the system.

Compared to implanting the electrode, connecting the system is child's play:

1. While you're under general anesthesia, your surgeon makes a small incision near your collarbone and inserts the implantable pulse generator (IPG) in a pocket formed under the skin.

2. Next, he runs a small wire from the IPG under the skin up your neck and behind your ear to connect the IPG to the DBS lead in your scalp.

3. Finally, your surgeon closes the incision with stitches or staples.

Hospitalization for DBS surgery is usually two to three days. For more complicated surgeries (when post-surgery confusion, infections, or other complications occur), the stay may be longer. In most cases, however, recovery is a matter of resting for a number of reasons: to get past the emotional and physical exhaustion that can be a part of any surgery; to rest after the possible slight headache (because of the helmet apparatus); and, in some cases, to reduce the mild confusion. Most DBS patients are able to leave the hospital the morning following the procedure.

Most routine postoperative conditions clear up after the first day. The stitches or staples in your scalp will be removed by your doctor a week or so after your discharge. The IPG (battery pack), which is usually implanted two to four weeks later, will be visible as a slight bump in your chest (especially if you're slender), but you don't feel the wires or apparatus as they work.

Programming DBS into Your Life

Surgery of any type takes a lot out of you. There's stress and anxiety from anticipating the procedure, exhaustion from the procedure itself, and suspense and concern about whether it worked, whether it was worth the trouble. This section helps you anticipate your life after your DBS surgery.

Changes you can expect

Following DBS surgery, your neurologist determines the best time to begin reducing your medication. But first, your neurostimulator must be programmed. This process may take one long session *(initial programming session)* and several outpatient visits, because just as you have unique responses to medication, you may have unique responses to the stimulator.

You may not realize the benefits of DBS for weeks or even months, although most people experience some effects the same day the unit is programmed.

> Tremors and dyskinesias are usually the first symptoms to respond. Be patient as your doctor works with you to balance the settings on your stimulator with your medication regimen.

During this sometimes-exasperating process, you may have some temporary discomfort, such as minor shocks or muscle spasms. These symptoms are related to adjusting and programming the neurostimulator and should be brief. Before you leave the office after a programming/adjustment session, your doctor may want you to wait an hour or so, just to be sure you're okay with the new settings.

Warning signs you need to heed

Although you may experience some discomfort and unusual symptoms as your neurostimulator is programmed, let your doctor know whether you experience any of the following symptoms after implantation or between programming sessions:

- Shocks or tingling sensations

- Numbness or spasms, especially in the face or hands

- Impaired balance or dizziness

- Slurred speech

- Blurred or double vision

- Depression

- Dykinesia-like movement

As you go about your normal routine, take these precautions:

- Ask for a hand-check when you go through security while traveling. If the electromagnetic field of the security equipment causes your stimulator to shut down, you can turn it back on with a handheld remote. Not to worry: Airport security personnel are accustomed to travelers who have implants such as a defibrillator or pacemaker.

- If you play sports, carefully rethink any high-level contact sports like basketball. Repeated direct blows to the implant or connections can cause harm or the need for replacement.

- At home, try to stay away from microwave ovens (while they're in use) and be aware of the magnetic strip that keeps the refrigerator door shut. Swiping it near your chest may inadvertently turn off your neurostimulator.

- Check with your neurologist before any doctor orders imaging tests such as an MRI or CT scan for you. The test may be perfectly safe for you, but it doesn't hurt to be sure.

- Other common warnings are provided in the patient-information manual you receive. Review them in detail with your treating physician or programming nurse.

Chapter 11

Considering Complementary and Alternative Medicine Therapies

In This Chapter

• Noting the distinctions: Alternative versus complementary therapies

• Grasping options for your mind and body

• Choosing the right CAM professional

• Spiriting the right approach

Medication and surgical procedures are only two of the options for treatment of your Parkinson's disease (PD) symptoms. Increasingly the healthcare profession is embracing the benefits of some complementary and alternative medical treatments.

This chapter helps you understand the differences between complementary and alternative therapies so you can sort through the various options and weigh the potential benefits of each. It also helps put you in touch with reputable practitioners if you decide to expand your treatment plan.

Don't underestimate the importance of diet and exercise to your success in managing your PD symptoms. These topics are so vital that they get their own discussion (see Chapter 12). In this chapter, though, we look at therapies you may have heard of but never considered as viable complements or alternatives to the conventional plan you expect your doctor to recommend.

What's in a Name? CAM Therapies Defined

Techniques, medicines, and therapies that take a holistic (mind, body, and spirit) and unconventional approach to the treatment of disease are often called *complementary* or *alternative medicine* (CAM) therapy.

Alternative medicine usually refers to approaches (yoga, T'ai Chi, acupuncture, special herbal remedies, diets, and the like) that aren't standard in Western society but are quite common in Eastern societies.

Complementary therapies, on the other hand, include techniques and approaches (physical, occupational, and speech therapy; modifications to diet; regular exercise, and such) that are more familiar to Western societies.

Alternative treatments often *replace* more convention-al treatments, and complementary therapies *augment* conventional methods.

Although alternative and complementary treatments may work in tandem with more traditional medical treatment, they usually haven't passed (or even been required to pass) the rigorous, scientific, evidence-based tests that conventional medicines and treatments must navigate for the Food and Drug Administration's (FDA) approval.

However, in 1998 the National Institutes of Health (NIH) established the National Center for Complemen-tary and Alternative Medicine (NCCAM) because of

- The growing popularity of alternative and complementary therapies.

- The need for establishing standards for practitioners.

- The need for a respected resource for validating information and conducting research on their benefits.

NCCAM focuses on four key areas:

- Research

- Training and career development for researchers working on projects related to alternative or complementary treatments

- Public outreach and education

- Integration of CAM treatments with conventional medicine

You can find information about specific therapies on the NCCAM Web site www.nccam.nih.gov or by calling (888)644-6226.

Before you consider any alternative or complementary therapy, talk with your neurologist and make sure the therapy is from a licensed, certified practitioner. (See the section "Finding the Best Practitioner" later in this chapter for tips on determining the right practitioners.)

The following section explores the major categories of CAM treatments available today.

Debunking the myths about treating PD

PD treatment has a number of urban myths that surface from time to time about what does and doesn't work. Often these falsehoods are from credible sources (such as members of your support group or even articles in respected, usually trustworthy publications). The Internet is another prime source for such rumors. For these reasons, remember to seek and confirm information by asking questions of your doctor or other trusted healthcare professionals (such as your pharmacist). And use only reliable PD information resources, such as those listed in Appendix B.

The following are some of the more prevalent myths floating around:

• Levodopa is toxic. (Actually it's been working for PWP for over 40 years.)

• Levodopa will stop working after a while. (No, but symptoms may escalate, causing you to need stronger, more frequent dosing.)

• You die from PD. (How you're going to die is as much a mystery now as it was before you were diagnosed—could be a car accident, lightening, a heart attack, and so on.)

• You're definitely going to be in a wheelchair. (Keep in mind that PD is unique to every person. Your chances of being in a wheel-chair are probably higher than some PWPs and far lower than others'.)

• You're definitely going to be demented—a vegetable. (PD has no definites. As for being a vegetable? Just focus on eating vegetables and stop predicting the future.)

• My children will have PD. (Go back and read Chapter 3—right now.)

• You can't eat proteins while taking levodopa. (Ah, the protein myth—see the section "The protein factor" later in this chapter. Meanwhile, eat your protein.)

• Surgery doesn't work for PD. (Right, it may not work for some people, but it does work in combination with prescription medications for many others, and you may be one of them.)

• You can cure PD with alternative therapies such as glutathione and nicotinamide adenine dinucleotide, NADH. (We've said it before and we'll say it again—PD doesn't have a cure yet.)

• And our personal favorite: You can cure PD with foot massage. (We're not even going to comment on that one.)

As you can see, each myth has a little bit of truth. Remember, somewhere along the way you were told: If something sounds too good to be true, it's probably not true. So when someone tries to sell you the snake-oil-of-a-cure, or a concoction that reverses symptoms, or a plan that halts PD's progression, just walk away. Your best weapons against this web of half-truths? Be informed, keep up with new research, and ask questions.

Introducing Your Options

The concept of any therapy other than traditional medical methods (medications and surgery) may be new to you. And one of the beauties of reading up on these various CAM options before you talk to your doctor about them is that you can do so in the privacy of your own home.

In this section, we introduce you to several of the more prevalent therapies. Before taking any action, though, be sure you discuss with your neurologist the potential of such therapies for helping your PD symptoms. (Then again, maybe your neurologist has suggested one or more of these techniques, and you're reading this section because you [wisely] want to get a better idea of just what you're in for.)

East treats West: Acupuncture and other traditional Chinese medicine

For centuries Western medical experts considered Eastern medical techniques to be experimental at best and quackery at worst. But much of that attitude has changed dramatically in the last decade. Traditional Chinese Medicine (TCM) is founded on the concept of *qi* (or *chi*), when the person's natural flow of energy is in balance. This system includes forms (such as exercise, herbal remedies, acupuncture, and massage) that work with identified energy points in the body.

Perhaps the most familiar TCM is acupuncture. This therapy usually requires a series of appointments by a trained and licensed therapist who inserts sterile needles (about the size of a human hair) into a part of the body believed to affect the area needing treatment. Although acupuncture has not been shown to relieve PD symptoms, it may help persons with Parkinson's (PWP) who experience cramping, stiffness, pain, or sleep disturbances.

In 1997, the NIH noted the increased use of acupuncture by a growing number of physicians and other medical professionals in the United States for relief or prevention of pain.

Ohhh! Ahhh! Experiencing body-based CAM therapies

Treatments that manipulate or move various parts of the body (such as muscles and joints) are considered body-based CAM therapies. Major examples of this category are chiropractic and osteopathic therapy and body massages.

Chiropractic and osteopathic therapy

Chiropractors focus on the structure of the body as it relates to the function, preservation, or restoration of various parts. ***Note:*** In chiropractic literature you may find some poorly defined theories that relate PD to previous head and neck traumas, which then suggest neck manipulations to treat (and cure!) the disease. Given that these assumptions are criticized even within the chiropractic profession, the role of chiropractic therapy in PD is unknown at this time.

Osteopathic medicine is a more-conventional medical system based on the principle that all the body's systems work together. When one system is affected, then other systems are likely to be affected as well. The hands-on techniques of some osteopaths to manipulate various body parts are considered a CAM therapy.

Massage

Many people associate massages with a ritzy spa or salon. But many medical professionals view regular massage therapy by a trained and certified therapist an important complement to conventional medical care. Massage can help relieve some of the stiffness and muscle contractions common in PD by

- Increasing blood supply to the muscles.

- Increasing range of motion.

- Stretching the muscles for greater flexibility.

The bonus to these physical benefits is the mental payoff: reduced stress and anxiety. You and your care partner may find that regular sessions with a massage therapist are a great way to relieve stress, build a sense of well being and calm, and improve circulation.

Massage is also a good form of relaxation. Under the right circumstances, it offers an environment conducive to meditation and centering. See the next section, "Exploring mind and body options to relieve tension, stress, and anxiety," for more about these benefits. You can also check out *Massage For Dummies* by Steve Capellini and Michel Van Welden (Wiley) for more info.

Therapeutic massage and other CAM therapies may be covered by your insurance if your doctor prescribes them as medically necessary.

Exploring mind and body options to relieve tension, stress, and anxiety

Mind and body therapies rely on the mind's ability to influence physical function and symptoms. They include meditation, creative outlets (as in music, art, or dance), and so on.

Employing relaxation and meditation techniques
Living with a chronic and progressive illness takes a lot out of you. Combine that reality with life's thousand other pressures (like work, relationships, financial security, crime, the weather, and such) and you have a prescription for stress. So when you have PD, finding ways to eliminate tension from your mind and body makes especially good sense.

You can have planned relaxation without going anywhere, hiring anyone, or paying any money. It's a simple matter of finding a quiet place to focus totally on you for at least 15 minutes twice a day. At the end of that time, close your eyes, hum a mantra, or sit cross-legged on a pillow—it's totally up to you.

Start by being aware of your *physical* tensions. Slowly and softly breathe in and out as you relax each muscle group one at a time: forehead, neck, shoulders, arms, hands, fingers, torso, hips, thighs, calves, ankles, feet, and finally toes. As you become more aware of your body relaxing, you have a better idea of where you tend to store that stress and tension (for example in the neck and shoulders, the fingers, or perhaps the jaw). Soon you'll be able to consciously relax those areas beyond your planned relaxation sessions.

Another tool is meditation, which you can use when your tension is not only physical but also mental and emotional. It can take many forms; consider the mantra-chanting practice of Zen meditation or the visualization techniques that follow recorded prompts to imagine (visualize) a calm, peaceful setting.

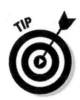

If you've never tried meditation, the Mayo Clinic recommends these tips to help you get started:

- Select a form of meditation that fits your lifestyle and daily routine and works with your fundamental beliefs.

- Set aside the time. If 15 minutes twice a day seems too much, start with 5 minutes and work your way up to longer sessions.

292

- Forgive your slips. If your mind wanders, recognize it. Then come back to your focus on relaxing and calming your mind, body, and spirit.

- Experiment until you find the timing and method that works best for you.

In combination with relaxation, meditation can reduce stress for mind and body. But, like all complementary and alternative practices, meditation should supplement—not replace—your doctor's traditional therapies.

Getting in touch with your creative side
Quilting. Woodworking. Gardening. Knitting. Playing an instrument. Dancing—by yourself or in a group. Writing poetry or stories. Journaling. Everyone has a creative side. And, as one sage said, "If something is worth doing, it'3 worth doing badly." You may not be Picasso or Mozart but you can find pleasure in creating something unique. Who knew that such pleasure could be good therapy as well?

At the 2006 World Parkinson Congress in Washington DC, one of the most popular areas was a wonderful art exhibition by dozens of PWP. To supplement the display, there were delightful performances by musicians, poets, story-tellers, and others. Some of the work was good enough to be in a fine gallery or shop, but the real beauty was in the obvious joy and delight of the artist in creating it. To see examples of the exhibit, go to www.pdcreativity.org.

Take these steps to get your creative side in gear:

- Find a new or return to a former hobby, art, or craft that appeals to you. Establish a regular time to pursue it—an hour every evening or once or twice a week if time is tight.

- Consider taking lessons at a local art center, community center, or shop. You can enjoy the dual therapy of creativity plus socialization.

Letting those creative juices flow isn't about being good. It's about finding pleasure, escape,

> and relief from the daily grind of managing your PD symptoms. Just say "Ahhh!"

Staying active via alternative exercise

Postural instability (the loss or impairment of your natural ability to hold yourself upright and maintain balance) can be a major problem for PWP. The greatest danger, of course, is falling. But a close second is the fear of falling that causes you to overcompensate for these off-balance positions, further jeopardizing your stability. One of the benefits of regular physical activity is realizing that alignment, stability, and balance are vital to our overall well being and independence.

For PWP, Eastern exercise programs may be as beneficial, if not more so, than the traditional, strenuous Western types. Eastern exercise therapies tend to be performed slowly and focus on stretching motions that can enhance flexibility. These Eastern methods aren't for everyone, but if you haven't been off the couch and gotten real exercise in a while, you may want to consider this variation.

Check with your doctor before beginning any exercise program—conventional or alternative.

T'ai Chi

This ancient, low-impact Chinese exercise combines measured breathing with slow, dance-like movements that develop flexibility, enhance cardiovascular well being, and improve balance. Although books and instructional visual aids are available, the best way to get started is by working with a trained professional to understand the proper moves and breathing combinations. Check with your local community center, senior center, or health club for classes in your area. T'ai Chi For Dummies by Therese Iknoian (Wiley) can provide a solid introduction.

Yoga

Another exercise program that incorporates stretching and balancing exercises in a slow, rhythmic pattern of movement is yoga. Forget the painful-looking, pretzel-like positions you may have seen on television or in movies. Yoga—properly done—combines stretching with breathing and meditation to achieve a greater sense of physical, mental, and spiritual balance.

As with T'ai Chi, yoga classes have levels from beginner to advanced and different styles of teaching. For example, some instructors focus more on the physical movement; others distribute the focus between the physical, breathing, and mind exercises.

If possible, find an instructor who can and will modify the traditional yoga positions and movements to accommodate your limitations. For example, if getting up and down from a mat is difficult, perhaps you can do a modified version of the movements while sitting in a chair. *Yoga For Dummies* by Georg Feuerstein and Larry Payne (Wiley) is a great reference for beginners.

Delving into dietary, protein, enzyme, and vitamin options

Although Chapter 12 has a detailed discussion of diet and exercise, the subject of complementary therapies also involves dietary issues. Because each person plays an active, participatory role in such therapies, this section provides information about CAM diets and diet supplements.

Diet—The usual rules apply

You know the drill. With or without PD, a healthy lifestyle includes a diet rich in fruits and vegetables but low in sugar, fats, and highly processed foods (*white* foods like white bread, white flour, white rice, and such). You also want to avoid foods that have been exposed to pesticides and other toxins. (Stick with organic fruits and vegetables even though they're more expensive—you're worth it!) As we mention in Chapter 2, overexposure to pesticides and herbicides (common in nonorganic farming) may be a contributing factor in the onset of PD. For additional help, consider asking your doctor to recommend a trained nutritionist.

This professional may suggest a diet high in antioxidants (green leafy vegetables and the like) because ongoing studies indicate that such a diet may be beneficial for PWPs. Another diet-specific concern is whether you're getting enough calcium (osteoporosis leads to softer bones, which lead to breaks from falls). Finally, studies have shown that the intake of protein in combination with antiparkinsonian meds can be a problem for some PWP. For more on the protein factor, see the next section.

The protein factor

A common PD myth is that protein in a PWP's diet is not good. Although you certainly don't want to remove protein from your diet, your doctor or nutritionist may recommend that you limit protein intake to particular meals and take your anti-PD meds (in particular levodopa/Sinemet) on an empty stomach.

As your PD progresses, you may experience the on-off phenomenon (your meds start to wear off sooner and symptoms reappear more rapidly between doses) that's common among PWP who've taken Sinemet for several years. Some studies indicate that diets rich in protein may negatively affect the brain's ability to absorb Sinemet if meals and dosing aren't properly coordinated. In fact, levodopa is an amino acid (the building block of every protein); a high protein intake at the same time of your medication dose may compete with the absorption of your precious medications. Taking levodopa 30 to 45 minutes before meals can avoid the problem.

CoQ10 and other over-the-counter supplements
CoQ10 (coenzyme Q10) is naturally produced by the body, but it decreases with age and in people with certain chronic conditions such as PD. Available as a dietary supplement, this enzyme may slow the progression of PD for some PWP.

In 2006 the NIH announced plans to enroll recently diagnosed and early-stage PWP in a study to determine whether exceptionally high doses of this over-the-counter (OTC) enzyme may indeed affect the progression of PD. "We're looking for the aspirin of Parkinson's disease," stated Diane Murphy, head of Parkinson's research at NIH. Although some patients already take CoQ10 (with the guidance of their neurologist, we hope), the NIH dosing plan is much higher than the recommended OTC dose.

Also under study are minocycline (an anti-inflammation antibiotic available only by prescription), and creatine, an energy-boosting dietary supplement. The fact that the federal government and medical community continue to sponsor such studies is a clear indication of their willingness to consider the possibility that PD may be better managed with the use of a combination of therapies rather than a single magic bullet.

Vitamin supplements

Taking vitamins that maintain your recommended daily levels is important for PWP. For example, a good multivitamin—one that includes the key B vitamins that are so important for brain and nerve health—is a good choice. Calcium with vitamin D helps prevent osteoporosis, which is a common concern for PWP, and calcium with magnesium can play a role in relieving muscle cramps. After running some standard blood tests, your doctor may make specific recommendations. Be sure to ask your doctor about continuing the vitamins and supplements you used before your diagnosis and about adding new ones.

Several studies have looked at vitamin E as a way to prevent the onset of PD or slow its progression. The most important was the DATATOP study, a ten-year controlled trial that found no benefit in slowing or improving the disease with the use of very high doses of vitamin E. Indeed, a recent report in the American Academy of Neurology's journal stated: "Vitamin E is probably ineffective in the treatment of PD." Moreover a recent analysis of medical literature warned that high-dosage vitamin E supplementation may actually increase mortality. In other words, too much of a good thing may not be a good thing.

On the other hand, scientists have found some protective qualities in the vitamin E in foods such as green leafy veggies, whole grains, and nuts. Mahyar Etminan, a lead researcher for the Centre for Clinical Epidemiology and Evaluation at Vancouver Hospital in Canada cautions that "this is an interesting hypothesis, but it needs to be validated." Of course, eating a diet rich in natural sources of vitamin E is always a good idea for your overall health.

In general, no regimen of vitamins has shown the ability to reduce or control PD symptoms. However, because one theory about the cause of PD (see Chapter 2) involves the oxidation of free radicals, it is possible that anti-oxidants (like vitamins C and E) may reduce the levels of these free radicals and, therefore, provide some benefit.

Interestingly, a trial that combined vitamin C and E supplements in people with early PD showed a delayed need for drug therapy (L-dopa) by an average of two and a half years. However, more studies are needed to confirm these findings. Similarly, because PWP can be prone to bone loss, your doctor may prescribe (especially for women patients) a calcium supplement or a prescription medication for preserving bone mass. See *Osteoporosis For Dummies* by Carolyn Riester

O'Connor and Sharon Perkins (Wiley) for more about this connection.

Finding the Best Practitioner

Keeping in mind that managing PD over the long haul is a team effort, be sure you talk to your neurologist about the potential benefits and pitfalls of alternative or complementary therapies you're considering. Your doctor may take a "no harm, no foul" attitude and not actually support the idea. Or she may suggest specific therapies for you to try or avoid.

Adding CAM therapy to your PD management plan requires you to carefully choose the person who'll administer that therapy. The following tips can help you in that search:

• If your neurologist endorses the idea, ask for recommendations.

• Be sure this person has received training from a respected source and passed the exams necessary to earn the appropriate degree or license.

• Acupuncturists and herbalists specializing in the use of herbs as medicine should be licensed.

Consider adapting the checklist for finding a neurologist (we provide this in Chapter 4) to guide your choice of alternative medicine practitioners.

After you've selected a practitioner, you still have a number of questions. On your first visit, ask:

- What benefits can I expect from this therapy?

- What are the risks associated with the treatment?

- Does it have any special benefits or risks related to my PD?

- What are the side effects?

- How many sessions or how long will I need to have the treatment to achieve the expected results?

- Does this treatment have any conditions that are contraindicated (to be avoided)?

- What is the cost per session?

- Will insurance pay?

You're not married to a specific practitioner. If you're uncomfortable with the treatment or the practitioner as the sessions proceed, then stop and talk the problem out. If you aren't satisfied with the response, move on.

Considering Your Approach to Life: It Too Can Help ... or Hinder

You know the difference between the eternal pessimist (who always expects the worst) and the forever optimist (who's over the top, always anticipating the best). Somewhere in the middle is the realist (as well as a bit of an idealist, philosopher, and activist) who accepts that bad things do indeed happen to good people. This person faces adversity and then looks for ways to get life back on track.

Celebrities like Lance Armstrong, Christopher and Dana Reeve, Michael J. Fox, Muhammad Ali, and others come to mind. But chances are good that you know people within your circle of family, friends, and co-workers who also fit this positive profile. As a PWP, you're going to benefit most from this glass-half-full- and-things-could-be- a-lot-worse philosophy.

Three characteristics that most survivor-types have in common are

- A *positive* attitude.

- The ability to laugh even at the unfairness of life.

- A spiritual core that's as well-tended as their physical or mental health.

The way you approach life—and all its joys and adversities—can play an enormous role in how successfully you live that life. The very fact that you bought this book and are reading it tells us that you're a survivor and a fighter. Our message to you is that we're right here with information and ideas that can help you successfully find ways to live a full and fulfilling life in spite of having PD.

The therapeutic power of positive thinking

Life has no guarantees. But a lot of people live life more fully by rolling with the punches and taking a positive, can-do approach.

So, how do you deal with a diagnosis like PD? How do you face the progressive symptoms and side effects of the medicines? Believe it or not, the one factor that remains in your control throughout this journey is your attitude. You can expect the worst or you can fight back by choosing to live life fully and positively—as if you had never heard that diagnosis.

As a matter of fact, for some people the diagnosis creates this shift in attitude. Discovering that they have PD turns their world upside down, so now they focus more intently on the positives. The realization that life is finite after all can be a real turning point for you—if it comes with the determination to live every day to the fullest. (And if your faith tells you that God doesn't test you more than you can endure, then you can start believing that higher opinion *and* start honing those survival capabilities!)

Laughter—Still the best medicine

Face it: When you laugh, you feel better. Your outlook improves—if only momentarily. You may even feel better physically. Consider the angry, depressed man who had just gone through brain surgery. He told his wife he didn't want any visitors. But when she ran into several close friends at the elevator and told them, "Not today," the friends still insisted. "We'll only stay a moment," they promised. Within moments the woman heard the welcome sound of laughter—her husband's. As the visit went on and the friends worked their magic, that laughter couldn't be repressed.

Open up to life—Physically, mentally, and spiritually

When you face a chronic and progressive illness day after day, you understandably have times when you just want to burrow under the covers and hope it all goes away. Resist that temptation!

Because we address your physical and mental well being throughout this book, this section looks at one other dimension, your spiritual needs, and how meeting those needs can enhance your life.

Spirituality is that core inside you where your sense of well being and survival reside. For some people, organized rituals of religion can be a part of this core, but rituals can't be all of it; for other people, rituals and religion play no part at all.

Your spiritual core is also where you store your self-identity. Your body may shake and twist and your mind may play tricks with your memory and concentration, but your spirit is still there. A relative of a PWP who was in the later stages said it well: "I just believe that he's still in there somewhere, that his spirit is still aware and fighting to let us know."

Like your PD, spirituality is different for every individual. But one way to begin focusing on your spiritual well-being is by using your senses to their full effect. Consider the following suggestions:

- Listen—to a sermon, an inspirational reading, a concert, water flowing, wind in the trees, rain on the roof, your innermost hopes and dreams

- Look—at the people who surround you, love you, and care for you

- Touch—by taking a friend's hand; petting a dog or cat; hugging a loved one; stroking a leaf, a rock, a child's hair

- Smell—freshly cut grass, an autumn fire, cookies straight from the oven

- Taste—the bitter as well as the sweet

- Savor—the unique tastes, sounds, sights, scents, and feelings that form the wonders of your life

Tapping into your spiritual side takes the same focused effort as your physical and mental needs. And your willingness to push yourself on all three levels can pay off in ways you never thought possible.

Chapter 12

The Key Roles of Diet and Exercise

In This Chapter

- Eating to live versus living to eat

- Improving mobility through exercise and activity

- Getting (and staying) physical

- Empowering the mind and spirit

You've heard it since you were a child—eat right and exercise! But, for people with Parkinson's (PWP) and their care partners, the importance of proper diet and a regular program of exercise can't be overemphasized. The benefits go well beyond physical fitness to bring relief from the general stresses of living with a chronic, progressive disease. In addition, a good diet and regular exercise help fight off the anxiety and depression that can accompany Parkinson's disease (PD). With or without PD, you owe it to yourself to be as fit—physically, mentally and spiritually—as possible. How else are you going to participate fully in life?

In this chapter we show you that good health isn't about training for a marathon or depriving yourself of foods you love. It's about making the choices that give you the best chance of living well and pursuing the pleasures of your life for many years—in spite of PD.

The Joy of Good Food—Diet and Nutrition

According to the National Institute of Aging, the combined effects of not making the right food choices and not being physically active make up the second largest underlying cause of death (behind smoking) in the United States. Often the element most absent from the diets of Americans is *nutrition,* foods that provide the proteins, carbohydrates, vitamins, minerals, hydration, fiber, and—yes—fats that the body needs to operate at its best. Add to that fact that PD medications and symptoms can significantly reduce the pleasures of eating, and you have a situation ripe for disaster.

This section isn't about losing that extra twenty pounds; it's about making the best food and nutrition choices to maintain optimal health as you fight the progression of PD.

Balance is the key

As a PWP, you have to perform a real balancing act when it comes to your diet. Along with the ready-made factors that impact nutrition and diet (like age, gender, and physical fitness), you have to deal with the nutritional sideshows of PD. For example, side effects of medications may include loss of appetite or even nausea. As your PD progresses, swallowing and constipation can become issues. And you may have side effects from medications for other chronic conditions, such as high blood pressure, diabetes, or arthritis.

Finding the proper balance between a healthy diet and these PD issues may require the help of a professional, so your neurologist may prescribe a consultation with a nutritionist or dietician as part of your treatment plan. If not, go ahead and ask him for a referral.

Keep in mind that timing the dosing of your medication (see Chapter 9) with meals is very important, especially for meals that include significant servings of protein. Protein—although essential for a balanced diet—can compete with the absorption of your antiparkinsonian meds. The usual recommendation is to take medication at least 30 minutes before meals unless you experience nausea or *dyskinesia* (uncontrolled twisting writhing motions) after taking your medications. If nausea is the problem, your doctor may recommend you take a low-protein snack, such as juice or saltines, with your meds. If dykinesia occurs, slowing the absorption by taking your anti-PD meds at mealtime may be exactly what you need. Be sure you and your doctor discuss the timing of meals and medications to offset this problem.

Banishing the bad and embracing the good-for-you foods

No doubt you've seen the food pyramid—which is now a bar grid—recommended by the U.S. Department of Agriculture. (See www.mypyramid.gov.) And you probably know you should hold your intake of fats and oils (not to mention desserts) to a minimum and spend most of your calories on fruits, veggies, whole grains, and dairy. (By the way, a banana split does not count in your fruit and dairy allowance!)

But this is your life, and presumably you're prepared to fight this PD that's parked like a tank in your designated space. A nutritionist or dietician can be a real help, showing you how to adapt your needs to your lifestyle. You tell her how you normally eat—on the run, in your car, at home standing at the kitchen counter, or seated with the family at the table, in fine restaurants, or fast-food joints. You reveal your food weaknesses—hate veggies, love bread, and such. Then the professional works with you to build a food plan that fits your lifestyle and your likes and dislikes.

Focus on these key issues when you start rearranging your pyramid:

• **Water, water, water!** Flavor it with a slice of lemon or a little fruit juice if you can't take it straight, but six to eight big glasses every day. (And, no, soda, coffee, and tea don't count.) Caffeine beverages may increase *diuresis* (your amount of urine output) and, as a result, cancel your efforts to hydrate your body. ***Note:*** Some studies have shown that caffeine may reduce the risk of PD for some people, so caffeine in moderation probably won't hurt—and may help.

• **Fiber** (whole-grain breads—not the mushy white stuff—brown rice, and whole-wheat pasta). In fact, stay away from white foods in general. Green leafy vegetables, whole grains, and nuts are rich natural sources of vitamin E that may have a protective effect against PD (see Chapter 11).

Whole grain breads must be refrigerated, but white bread isn't. (White bread is so devoid of actual nutrients that even bacteria won't eat it. That's a pretty good clue.)

- **Bone-strengthening nutrients (calcium, magnesium, and vitamins D and K).** Think dairy products and, believe it or not, exposure to sunlight (a vitamin D source). Also, regular exercise (we discuss this later) can help you keep bones strong, maintain balance, and prevent the falls so devastating for PWP.

Although your doctor may recommend adding supplements (such as a daily multivitamin, iron, or

316

> calcium pill) to your regular diet, the key word here is *supplement.* Such products are no substitute for a nutritionally balanced diet.

But good-for-you foods can actually be more delicious and easy to prepare than you imagined. One example is the fabulous fruit smoothie: Throw berries, half a banana, a cup of fat-free yogurt, and some ice cubes in a blender. Add a teaspoon of ground flax seed for fiber, turn the blender on high, pour the milkshake-like concoction into your car mug, and you're good to go (Smoothies are also great for preventing the constipation associated with PD medications.)

Food as celebration

If, like millions of Americans, you've fallen into a rut with the when, what, and where you eat, think about spicing those meals up. The following is our list of ideas for making meals more of a celebration than an afterthought:

• Choose your setting to match the menu, the mood, and the season—dining room, kitchen table, inside, outside; at home or at a sidewalk café.

• Set the table, even if it's just for one.

• Think *S.H.E.* when cooking at home—simple, healthy, and engaging.

• Try adding special (non-salt) seasonings and flavorings to spice up your food and make it more enjoyable.

• Be adventurous and try new dishes you've never tasted when eating out.

Request a soup spoon when ordering items like rice or small veggies (peas, corn, and such). A large spoon makes these foods easier to manage if you have a tremor.

• Savor food with all your senses—the vision of healthy food presented well; the smells, tastes, and textures; even the sounds of laughter and conversation interspersed with clinking dishes and glasses.

Food is life—and as a PWP, you understand the importance of celebrating every moment.

Use It or Lose It—The Healing Power of Exercise and Activity

Plenty of research backs up the fact that regular exercise can do wonders for your health. Consider that

- Exercising regularly boosts the power of neuro-transmittors in your brain to enhance your mood and your ability to see life in a more positive light.

- Exercise can relieve the muscle tension from your body's natural instinct to lock up in the face of challenges or battles.

- Exercise can enhance your self-image, which can lead to greater self-assurance and confidence, which can lead to a greater ability to deal with life's stresses.

Talk about a win-win!

In addition, PWP who exercise regularly seem to experience a milder and less-progressive disease process. In fact, exercise may be as good for brain function as it is for heart and weight factors. Recent laboratory experiments on animals have shown that physical exercise can potentially reduce the rate at which brain cells die. Further studies are under way to see whether regular exercise can actually slow the progression of PD.

Many exercise programs can benefit PWP. The Performance Centers of Wheaton Franciscan Healthcare in Milwaukee, Wisconsin designed the following exercises specifically to stretch and strengthen the key muscle groups for optimal flexibility and balance. Your doctor and physical therapist may fine-tune these exercises to match your specific needs, but this chapter gives you a good starting point. Begin the routine with the stretching exercises and repeat them during the cool-down period after the strengthening exercises.

The principles of a stretching/flexibility exercise program for PD are the same as those for sports-medicine rehabilitation:

- Listen to your body.

- Avoid joint pain during exercise.

- Forget the Vince Lombardi adage: No pain, no gain.

- Remember, for joint or other pain after exercise, "Ice is nice; hot is not."

Because PD frequently develops in a person's later years, other bone and joint conditions may already be present such as *osteoarthritis* (wearing of joints) and *osteoporsis* (thinning of the bones). So before you begin any exercise therapy, get the approval of your doctor and a prescription to work with a trained, experienced physical therapist.

A stretching program to enhance flexibility

The following exercises are designed to enhance your flexibility. With your doctor or physical therapist's initial guidance and ongoing monitoring, do the exercises every day, even twice a day.

If you also do strengthening exercises (such as the ones in the "A strengthening program to build muscle and stabilize joints" section later) or an aerobic activity, such as walking, bicycling, swimming, or working out on a treadmill, use these stretching exercises to warm up and cool down.

321

Stretching should be slow, smooth, and gentle. No bouncing allowed! And if it starts to hurt, listen to your body and ease up.

Neck stretches

Begin your routine by gently stretching the muscles in your neck, head, and shoulders.

The Chin Tuck

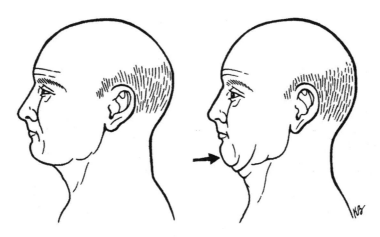

Figure 12-1: Chin Tuck

To perform the Chin Tuck:

1 Looking forward, tuck your chin by pulling it in—a little like a turtle (see Figure 12-1).

2 **Hold your chin in the tucked position for five seconds.**

3 **Untuck your chin and relax.**

Repeat this exercise five to ten times.

The Head Turn
To perform the Head Turn:

1. Looking straight ahead, slowly turn your head to the right until you're looking at the wall or view to your right (see Figure 12-2).

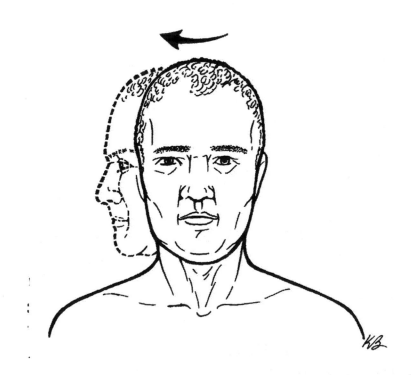

Figure 12-2: Head Turn

Don't force the movement; at first you may only be able to turn your head slightly to the right or left; with practice you'll become more flexible.

2. Hold the position for five seconds and return to center.

3. Repeat Steps 1 and 2, this time turning to your left.

Repeat this exercise five to ten times on each side.

The Head Tilt
To perform the Head Tilt:

1. Looking straight ahead, bend your head to the right as if to rest your head on your right shoulder (see Figure 12-3).

Don't raise your shoulder—let the stretch of your neck do the work.

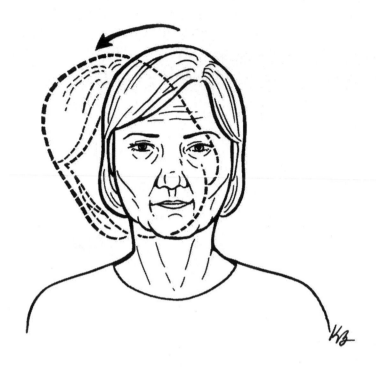

Figure 12-3: Head Tilt

2. Hold the position for five seconds, and raise your head back to straight ahead position.

3. Repeat Steps 1 and 2, this time bending to your left side.

Repeat this exercise five to ten times on each side.

The Shoulder Roll
To perform the Shoulder Roll:

1. **Standing tall and looking straight ahead, lift and roll both shoulders back in a circular motion five times (see Figure 12-4).**

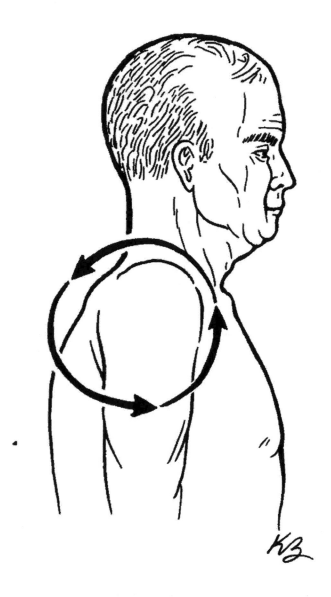

Figure 12-4: Shoulder Roll

2. **Relax.**

3. **Lift and roll shoulders forward in a circular motion five times.**

4. **Relax.**

Repeat the backward and forward rolls five to ten times each.

The Chest and Shoulder Stretch

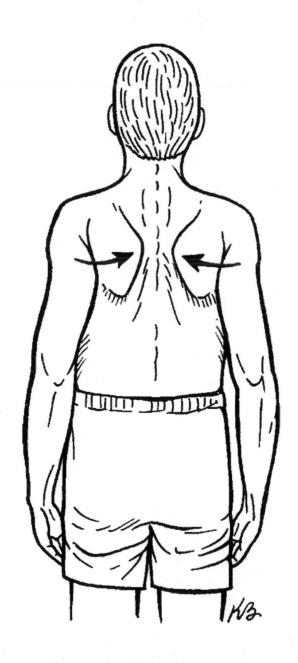

Figure 12-5: Chest and Shoulder Stretch

To perform the Chest and Shoulder Stretch:

1. **Standing tall and looking straight ahead with arms at your sides, pull your shoulder blades together (see Figure 12-5).**

2. **Hold for five seconds, and then relax.**

Repeat this exercise five to ten times.

Upper body stretches

Use the following stretches before and after your regular exercise routine to lengthen your muscles and prevent muscle pulls and tears.

The Posterior Shoulder Stretch
To perform the Posterior Shoulder Stretch:

1. **Reach your right arm across your chest, and place your right hand over your left shoulder (see Figure 12-6).**

2. **With your left hand, grasp your right elbow and apply light pressure to the elbow, moving your right arm closer to your chest.**

3. **Hold for five seconds, and return your arms to your sides.**

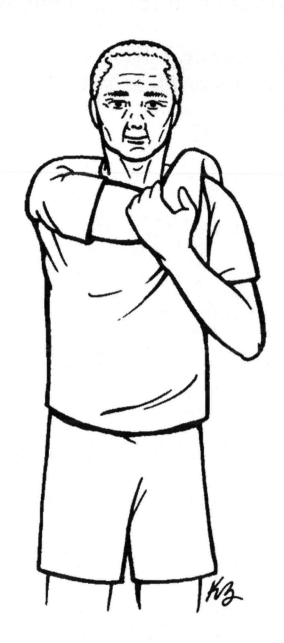

Figure 12-6: Posterior Shoulder Stretch

4. **Repeat Steps 1 through 3, this time stretching your left shoulder.**

Repeat this exercise five to ten times on each side.

The Anterior Shoulder Stretch

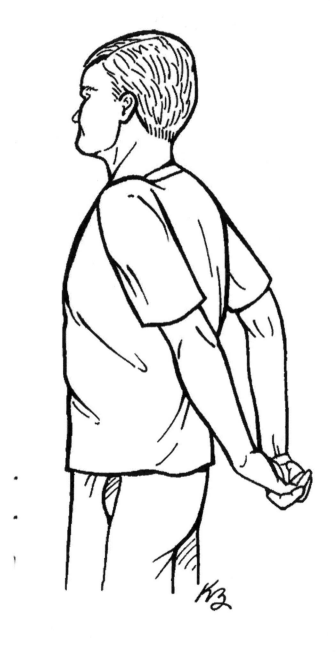

Figure 12-7: Anterior Shoulder Stretch

To perform the Anterior Shoulder Stretch:

1. **Reach behind your back and clasp your hands, interlocking your fingers and keeping your arms straight, with elbows turned in (see Figure 12-7).**

2. **Lift up your arms until you feel a stretch (not pain) in your shoulders and across your chest.**

3. **Hold your arms in the elevated position for five seconds.**

4. **Lower your hands, and relax.**

Repeat this exercise five to ten times.

The Posterior Shoulder Side Stretch
To perform the Posterior Shoulder Side Stretch:

1. **Raise your right arm above and behind your head, reaching toward your left shoulder (see Figure 12-8).**

2. **With your left hand, reach behind your head and pull your right elbow gently in toward your head.**

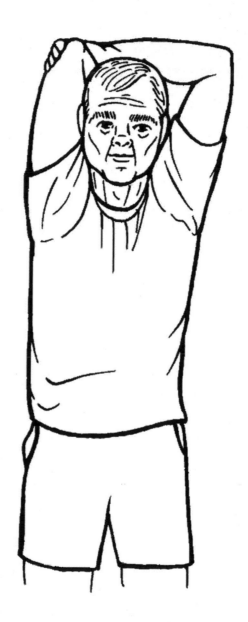

Figure 12-8: Posterior Shoulder Side Stretch

3. **Hold for five seconds and relax, returning your arms to your sides.**

332

4. Repeat Steps 1 through 3, this time stretching your left side.

Repeat this exercise five to ten times on each side.

The Wrist/Forearm Stretch
To perform the Wrist/Forearm Stretch:

1. Extend your right arm straight in front of you, fingers pointing toward the floor.

2. With your left hand, gently pull your fingers and hand down (see Figure 12-9a).

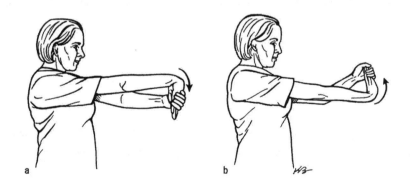

Figure 12-9: Wrist/Forearm Stretch

Your arm should remain extended.

3. Hold for five seconds, and then release your fingers.

4. Repeat Steps 2 and 3 five to ten times.

5. Flex your right wrist back so your fingers point to the ceiling.

6. With your left hand, gently press your fingers and palm back toward your forearm (see Figure 12-9b).

7. Hold for five seconds, and then release your fingers.

8. Repeat Steps 1 through 7, this time extending your left arm and stretching your left wrist and forearm.

Repeat this exercise five to ten times on each side.

Leg stretches
These stretches work on the hips, legs, knees, and ankles. As with any stretch exercise, they're good before and after your strengthening or aerobic routine to prevent muscle-strain tears and pulls.

The Hamstring Stretch
To perform the Hamstring Stretch:

1. Sitting on the floor with your right leg straight out in front of you, bend your left leg so the bottom of your left foot rests on the inner thigh of your extended right leg (see Figure 12-10).

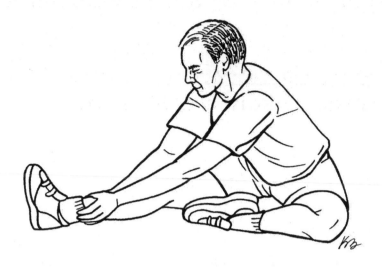

Figure 12-10: Hamstring Stretch

2. With your hands on your outstretched calf or ankle, slowly bend forward from the waist, keeping your back straight.

Don't bounce. Stretch only until you feel a mild (non-painful) stretching sensation in the back of your thigh.

3. Hold the stretch for five seconds, and then relax, releasing your calf or ankle and returning to the upright position.

4. Repeat Steps 1 through 3 five to ten times with your right leg.

5. Repeat Steps 1 through 4, this time extending your left leg and tucking your right leg.

Do five sets of five to ten repetitions each per side.

The Quadriceps Stretch
To perform the Quadriceps Stretch:

1 Standing beside a table, place your left hand on the table for balance.

2 Bending your right knee, grasp your ankle with your right hand and pull your foot backward toward your buttocks (see Figure 12-11).

3. Hold the stretch for five seconds and then relax, returning your right foot to the floor.

4. Repeat Steps 1 through 3 five to ten times.

5. Turn around (or move to the opposite side of the table) and repeat Steps 1 through 3, this time bending your left knee.

Do five sets of five to ten repetitions per side.

The Standing Gastroc Stretch
To perform the Standing Gastroc Stretch:

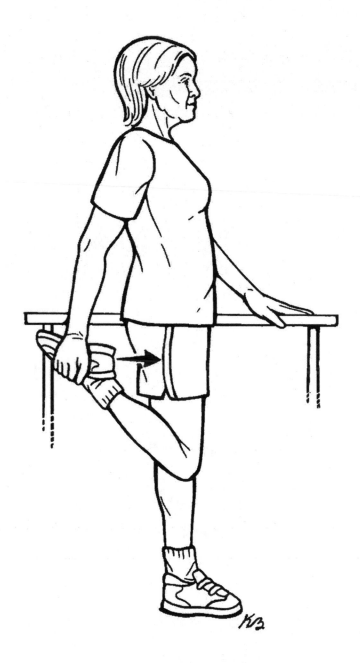

Figure 12-11: Quadriceps Stretch

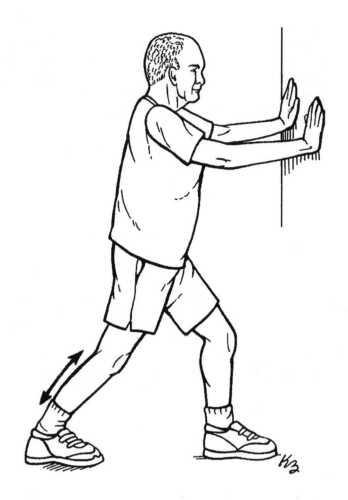

Figure 12-12: Standing Gastroc Stretch

You can also place a belt around your ankle and grasp it.

> Don't lean forward. Feel the stretch in the front of your thigh.

1. Standing about 2 feet from the wall, lean forward so flattened palms are against the wall.

2. Keeping your left foot planted, bend your left knee as you step backward with your right leg; lean forward into the wall until you feel a stretch in your right calf (see Figure 12-12).

Your right leg should remain straight, with your heel on the floor and your toes turned slightly outward.

3. Hold for five seconds and then relax, bringing your feet together.

4. Repeat Steps 1 through 3 five to ten times.

5. Repeat Steps 1 through 4, this time bending your right knee and stepping backward with your left leg.

Repeat this exercise five to ten times on each side.

The Inner Thigh (Groin) Stretch
To perform the Inner Thigh (Groin) Stretch:

1. Sitting on the floor, bend your knees so the soles of your feet face each other (see Figure 12-13).

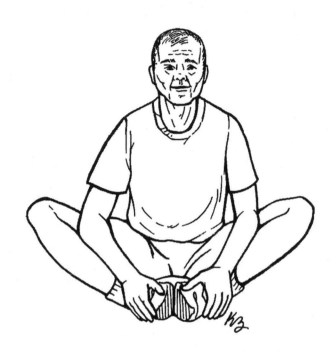

Figure 12-13: Inner Thigh (Groin) Stretch

2. Cup your hands around your toes, and gently press down on your thighs with your forearms until you feel a gentle stretch in your inner thighs.

Don't bounce your knees—stretch only until you feel a slight pulling sensation in your inner thigh.

3. Hold for five seconds, and then relax.

340

Repeat this exercise five to ten times.

Lower back stretches
The following stretches can protect your back from injury and help you maintain flexibility.

Knees to Chest
To perform the Knees to Chest Stretch:

1. **Lying on your back, slowly raise your right knee to your chest (see Figure 12-14).**

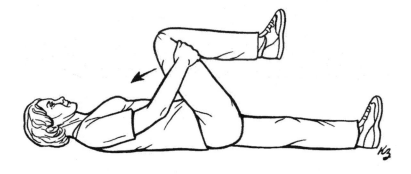

Figure 12-14: Knees to Chest

2. **Use your hands to hold your knee to your chest; you should feel the stretch in your lower back.**

3. **Hold this position for five seconds and then relax, returning your right leg to the floor.**

4. **Repeat Steps 1 through 3 five to ten times.**

5.   **Repeat Steps 1 through 4, this time bringing your left knee to your chest.**

Repeat this exercise five to ten times on each side.

Bridging
To perform the Bridging Stretch:

1.   **Lying on your back with your arms at your sides, bend your knees so your feet are flat on the floor (see Figure 12-15).**

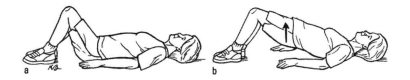

Figure 12-15: Bridging

2.   **Tightening your stomach muscles, slowly raise your buttocks until even with your knees.**

3.   **Hold this position for five seconds and then relax, lowering your buttocks to the floor.**

Repeat this exercise five to ten times.

Alternate Arm and Leg Lifts
To perform the Alternate Arm and Leg Lifts Stretch:

1. Lying on your stomach, extend your arms over your head.

2. Tightening your stomach muscles, simultaneously raise your *right* arm and your *left* leg 3 to 6 inches off the floor (see Figure 12-16).

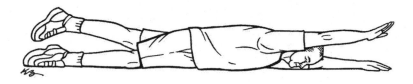

Figure 12-16: Alternate Arm and Leg Lifts

Keep both arms and both legs straight.

3. Hold this position for five seconds and then relax, returning both limbs to the floor.

4. Repeat Steps 1 through 3 five to ten times.

5. Repeat Steps 1 through 4, this time raising your *left* arm and *right* leg.

Repeat this exercise five to ten times on each side.

Standing Extension
To perform the Standing Extension Stretch:

1. **With both hands on your lower back, bend as far back as is comfortable (see Figure 12-17).**

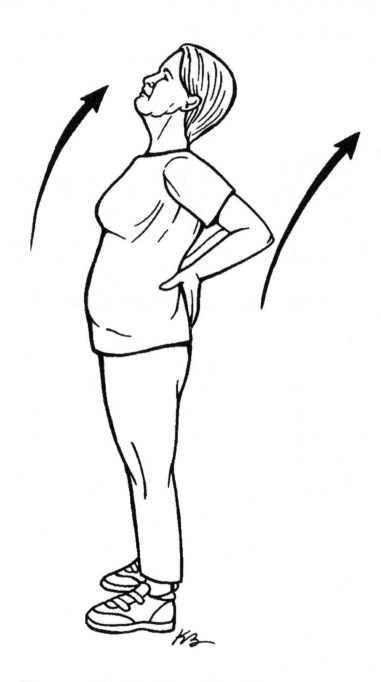

Figure 12-17: Standing Extension

2. **Hold this position for five seconds and then relax, straightening to the upright position.**

Repeat this exercise five to ten times.

A strengthening program to build muscle and stabilize joints

Although stretching is key to maintaining flexibility, don't ignore the benefits of strengthening your muscles—especially the muscles you need for maintaining balance and postural stability. You can perform the following shoulder and leg exercises three to five times a week to help maintain strength in these key areas.

Shoulder strengthening
The following exercises strengthen the shoulder area, especially the rotator cuff muscles (where your shoulder and arm connect). Your physical therapist can provide the stretchy exercise bands as well as help you adjust the tension and size to your needs. Or you can purchase a five-foot length of rubber tubing at a hardware store or athletic supply shop (they call it a *sports cord*). For some of the exercises, you also need a large bath towel to stabilize your arm.

Internal Rotation
To perform the Internal Rotation Exercise:

1. **Attach a band to a doorknob that's even with your elbow, and be sure the door is solidly shut.**

2. **Standing three feet from the door with your right side toward the door, grasp the band with your right hand, bending your arm at the elbow.**

3. **Place a rolled towel under your right arm, between your arm and right side of your body to stabilize your arm (see Figure 12-18a).**

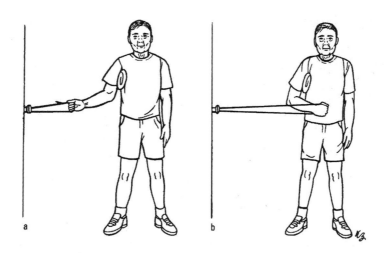

Figure 12-18: Internal Rotation

4. **Pull the band slowly across your body, rotating your arm and shoulder inward (see Figure 12-18b).**

5. **Slowly return your arm to its start position.**

6. **Repeat Steps 1 through 5 five to ten times.**

7. **Turn around so your left side is toward the door (move the towel under your left arm), and repeat Steps 1 through 5, this time extending your left arm.**

Repeat this exercise five to ten times.

External Rotation
To perform the External Rotation Exercise:

1. **Wrap the ends of a sports band around each hand.**

2. **Place a rolled towel under your right arm (between your arm and chest to stabilize your arm), and place your left hand on your left hip, keeping your right hand close by (see Figure 12-19a).**

3. **With your right hand, slowly pull the band across your body, rotating your arm and shoulder outward (see Figure 12-19b).**

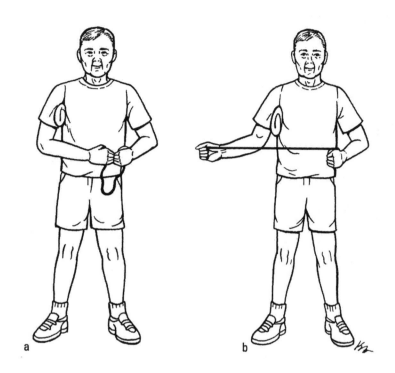

Figure 12-19: External Rotation

4. **Slowly return your arm to its start position.**

5. **Repeat Steps 1 through 4 five to ten times.**

6. **Repeat Steps 1 through 5, this time extending your left arm. (Don't forget to place the towel under your left arm.)**

Repeat this exercise five to ten times.

Extension Pull
To perform the Extension Pull Exercise:

1. **Attach a band to a doorknob that's even with your elbow, and be sure the door is solidly shut.**

2. **Stand facing the door (about 3 feet from the door) with the band in your right hand (see Figure 12-20a).**

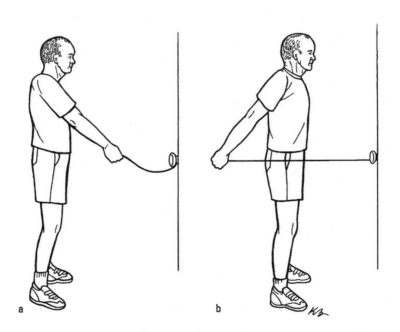

Figure 12-20: Extension Pull

3. Starting with your arm straight and forward, pull the band back by slowly lowering your straight-

ened arm until it's at your side (see Figure 12-20b).

4. Slowly return your arm to its start position.

5. Repeat Steps 1 through 4 five to ten times.

6. Repeat Steps 1 through 5, this time extending your left arm.

Repeat this exercise five to ten times.

Flexion

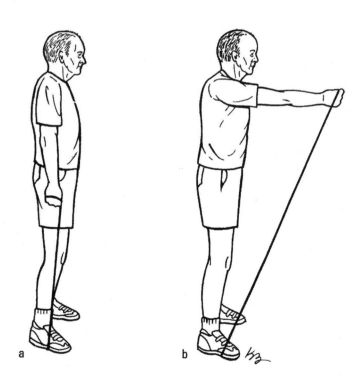

Figure 12-21: Flexion

To perform the Flexion Exercise:

1. **Place one end of an exercise band under your right foot and hold the other end in your right hand (see Figure 12-21a).**

2. **With your thumb on top of the band and your elbow straight, raise your right arm forward until it's level with your shoulder (see Figure 12-21b).**

3. **Slowly return your right arm to its start position.**

4. **Repeat Steps 1 through 3 ten times.**

5. **Repeat Steps 1 through 4, this time extending your left arm.**

Repeat this exercise five to ten times.

Horizontal Pull
To perform the Horizontal Pull Exercise:

1. **Hold the band with both hands at shoulder height (see Figure 12-22a).**

2. **With your hands close together, extend your arms out in front of you and slowly stretch the band out until your arms are wide open (see Figure 12-22b).**

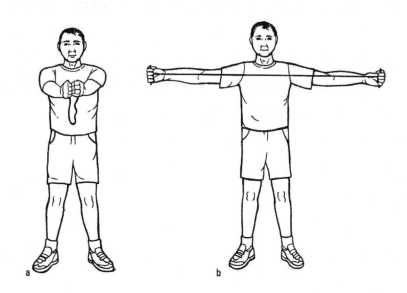

Figure 12-22: Horizontal Pull

3.   **Slowly bring your arms back together.**

Repeat this exercise five to ten times.

Leg strengthening

Your muscles are the stabilizers for your joints. Exercises that stretch and strengthen the muscles surrounding your hips, knees, and ankles can prevent injury and possibly improve balance. Perform the following exercises at least three times a week.

Straight Leg Raise
To perform the Straight Leg Raise Exercise:

1. Lying on your back, prop yourself up on your forearms, and slightly bend your left knee; keep your left foot flat on the floor.

2. Tightening your right leg's front thigh muscle, raise your right leg 8 to 10 inches from the floor (see Figure 12-23).

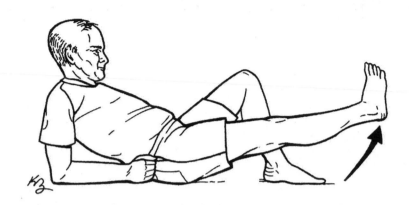

Figure 12-23: Straight Leg Raise

Keep the extended leg straight and knee locked as you perform the exercise.

3. Slowly return your right leg to the start position.

4. Repeat Steps 1 through 3 five to ten times.

5. Repeat Steps 1 through 4, this time bending your right leg and raising your left leg.

Repeat this exercise five to ten times.

Hip Abduction
To perform the Hip Abduction Exercise:

1 **Lie on your left side with both legs straight.**

2 **Slowly lift your right leg toward the ceiling to a comfortable height (at least 5 to 10 inches), keeping both legs straight (see Figure 12-24).**

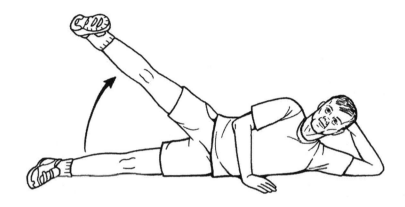

Figure 12-24: Hip Abduction

3 **Slowly lower your right leg.**

4 **Repeat Steps 1 through 3 ten times.**

5 **Turn to your right side and repeat Steps 1 through 4, this time lifting your left leg.**

Repeat this exercise five to ten times.

Hip Adduction
To perform the Hip Adduction Exercise:

1. **Lying on your right side with your right leg straight, bend your left leg at the knee so your left foot is flat on the floor in front of your right thigh or knee.**

2. **Keeping your right leg straight, raise your right leg off the ground 5 to 10 inches (see Figure 12-25).**

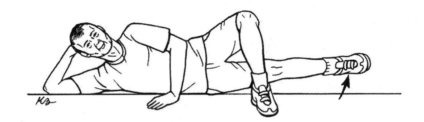

Figure 12-25: Hip Adduction

3. **Slowly lower your right leg to its start position.**

4. **Repeat Steps 1 through 3 five to ten times.**

5. **Turn to your left side and repeat Steps 1 through 4, this time lifting your left leg.**

Repeat this exercise five to ten times.

Hip Extension
To perform the Hip Extension Exercise:

1. **Lie on your stomach with both arms bent and under your chest.**

2. **With legs straight, and knees locked, tighten the muscle in your right thigh and lift your right leg 8 to 10 inches off the ground (see Figure 12-26).**

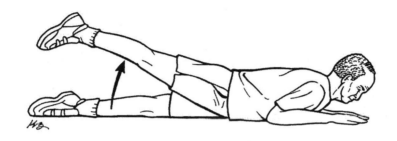

Figure 12-26: Hip Extension

3. **Slowly lower your leg back to the ground.**

4. **Repeat Steps 1 and 2, this time lifting your left leg.**

Repeat this exercise five to ten times.

Wall Slide
To perform the Wall Slide Exercise:

1. **Standing 12 to 16 inches from the wall and facing away from the wall with your feet shoulder-width apart, lean back against the wall.**

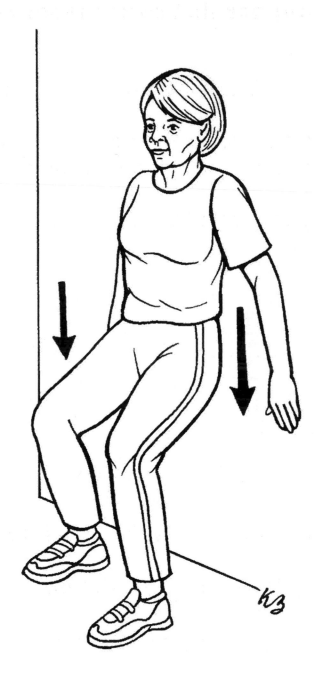

Figure 12-27: Wall Slide

2. **Slowly lower your buttocks toward the floor as far as you can, but no more than your**

thighs being parallel to the floor (see Figure 12-27).

3.   **Hold this position for five to ten seconds.**

4.   **Tighten your thigh muscles and slide back up to a standing/leaning position.**

Repeat this exercise five to ten times.

Toe Raise
To perform the Toe Raise Exercise:

1.   **Stand with both feet flat on the floor.**

2.   **Lift your heels and rise up on your toes (see Figure 12-28).**

3.   **Hold this position for five seconds.**

4.   **Lower your heels back to the floor.**

Repeat this exercise five to ten times.

Other exercise programs that can help

After you've mastered the stretches and exercises in the preceding sections, you may be ready for a program that's more challenging and yet specifically structured for PWP. Many national PD organizations consider regular exercise so essential that they've created a variety of programs and tools to help you get started. Some of these aids are listed below. For more options in programs and equipment, be sure to check out Chapter 23.

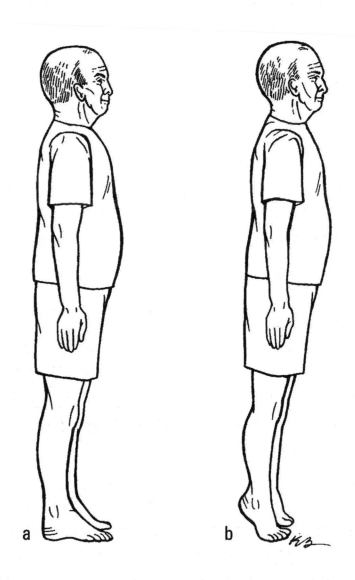

Figure 12-28: Toe Raise

Two programs available through the Parkinson's Disease Foundation (PDF) are:

- *Motivating Moves for People with Parkinson's:* In this program developed by movement specialist Janet Hamburg, participants sit while doing the exercises. The program is available in either VHS or DVD format.

- *The Exercise Program:* This tool by Dr. E. Richard Blonsky and a team of physical therapists specializing in rehabilitation therapy comes with audio instruction tapes and a binder with illustrated exercise cards.

Call 1-800-457-6676 for more information on either program.

The American Parkinson Disease Association (APDA) has free booklets entitled *Aquatic Exercises for Parkinson's Disease* and *Be Active: A Suggested Exercise Program for People with Parkinson's Disease.* For information, call 1-800-223-2732 or look online at www.apdaparkinson.org.

Structured exercise is important in maintaining flexibility and physical function, but equally important is maintaining an active lifestyle. Read on for ways that you can use daily physical activity to enhance your well being.

Beyond a Structured Exercise Program—PD and Physical Activity

Finding ways to redefine ourselves—especially following life-changing events such as career changes, retirement, the end of a relationship, or a diagnosis of PD—is not new to most adults. But when circumstances change the way we define our satisfaction and happiness, we either adapt or choose a less-than-satisfactory mindset, which may include depression and self-pity. Far better to work at rediscovering our identity with new resources for pleasure and purpose.

The saying "Quality trumps quantity in life" may not resonate for everyone. But if you have a PD diagnosis, then you have a choice: Bury your head in the sand or get out there and live each day to the fullest.

Enjoying recreation

Physical activity, or recreation (see how that word is really *recreation?*), differs from exercise because recreation usually provides an element of immediate pleasure, accomplishment, or revitalization that structured exercise may not. For example, if you garden, think about the pleasure of seeing the results of your hard work. In a similar way, biking and canoeing allow us to be physically active while taking in the fresh air and scenery.

But recreation goes beyond simple physical endeavors; it includes contact with other people and opening ourselves to new experiences and information. When we were kids, we called it *playing.* But adults can still play, even when they're facing grown-up stuff like PD.

Keeping up with routine roles and activities

Chances are good that you played multiple roles before getting the diagnosis of PD. Take a moment to list them: son/daughter, spouse/lover, friend/companion, parent/grandparent, employee/employer/co-worker, community leader/volunteer. How about the roles you played at home? Cook, gardener, decorator, financial manager, handyman/woman.

Ask yourself whether you think some of these roles are no longer possible. For example, do you think you can't keep up with your current job (see Chapter 16) or do you withdraw from social functions because you don't want pity from friends and family (see Chapter 15)? Maybe you don't cook anymore because the tremors make a mess. Or maybe you're afraid of making a mistake in the checkbook, so you've handed over the finances to your significant other.

Now take a good look at Chapters 2 and 3 to see whether you find a cause or symptom of PD that says you have to start peeling away pieces of your life and abandoning vital relationships. We'll wait.... Did you see it? Ah hah! We knew you wouldn't!

This is a good time for you to re-evaluate those activities you may have assumed were no longer possible—employment, volunteer work, and social activities, such as card playing, sports, and the like. The harder you work to maintain your normal routine and activities, the less likely your PD will dominate your life.

True, you may need to make some adjustments in physical activities to accommodate your PD. For example, you may find that sports requiring more lateral (side-to-side) movement, such as golf and ping pong, are easier for you. Or, if you were a marathon runner, think about race-walking or just plain walking. One PWP, Parky, biked over 42,000 miles in a ten-year period by switching to a recumbent three-wheel trike. (See www.inevergiveup.org. for more about his story.) His motto: "Let's take the PARK out of Parkinson's."

The point is that you do have choices and you can take charge instead of allowing assumptions to dictate your routine. Work with your doctor and other members of your professional health team to determine the right physical activities for you.

The same advice for physical activities applies to activities that engage you mentally and spiritually. This next section suggests ways to incorporate mental and spiritual activity into your daily life.

Exercises for the Mind and Spirit

Okay, you're exercising regularly and maintaining an active and productive lifestyle. Caring for the physical body is huge for you and for those people who make this journey with you. But be sure you give attention to the mind and spirit. What's happening inside your head? For that matter, what's going on with your care partner—that person (or persons) who's been with you from the moment you were diagnosed with PD?

In fact, many PWP develop apathy, a condition defined by

- Reduced interest and participation in routine activities

- Lack of initiative

- Difficulties in starting or sustaining an activity

- Lack of concern for events and people around them

In other words, the mind and spirit seem to simply give up.

Apathy in PD is more likely a direct consequence of *physiological* changes in the brain than a *psychological* reaction to the disability. As a result, this condition is different from the other psychiatric symptoms and personality changes associated with the disease (such as depression and anxiety—see Chapter 13). In addition, PD apathy can trigger major frustration for that person's care partner especially when the care partner sees that he's working harder at keeping the PWP active and involved than the PWP is.

Basically you can approach your life's uncertainties in two ways: Devote your efforts to worrying and trying to change the situation, or devote your energy toward living the most fulfilling life you can. Although you can't control the progression of your PD, you can control your choices:

- To exercise or not

- To remain engaged in the community or not

- To set a tone for your friends and family that you may have PD but it does not have you

- To wake up every morning and make good choices all over again or not

Choices for the person with PD

Just as proper diet and exercise are the best choices for maintaining your physical health, they're also your best weapons for maintaining the health of your mind and spirit. People who walk, bike, or run often report that they do their best thinking then; they're working out mental and emotional issues as well as physical ones.

These are some exercises you can make a part of your daily (or at least weekly) routine:

- Take time out for daily spiritual renewal (see Chapter 11). Meditate, pray, read inspirational books or poetry, take a walk, attend religious services—whatever gives you a sense of renewal.

- Challenge your mind. Work a crossword or Sudoku puzzle, play along with a TV game show (preferably one that actually requires some mental effort), read a book.

- Learn something new. Take a class at the local college or community center, ask a friend to teach you a craft or new sport, attend a lecture, watch a documentary. Then share your new ideas with someone else.

- Get involved in your community by taking an active role in a cause or organization that you think is important: the local library, a museum or historical site, national projects with local chapters (such as Habitat for Humanity).

- Create a legacy for your children and grandchildren. Write or record your family history, research the family tree, organize photo collections into albums that truly tell the story of your family's past.

- Partner with your partner to find activities you both can participate in and maintain the activities you both enjoyed before your diagnosis. Go to that play, that ballgame, that festival.

- Join a support group—preferably one for PWP—where you can interact with other people who fully understand the problems you and your care partner are facing.

- Accept that life with PD has no more certainty than life before PD. Turn to the *Bill of Rights for the Person Living with Parkinson's* in the front of this book. Tear it out, read it, and put it where you'll see and read it every day.

Choices for the PD care partner

As the care partner to someone living with PD, you also live with it. It affects your daily life in ways you had never imagined or planned for. A person in your shoes may want to abandon pieces of her own life to take care of the partner. And the most likely piece to fall by the wayside is your own physical health. You eat (or maybe don't eat!) as a reaction to your worries rather than as a source of nourishment. And when you add the responsibilities of caring for someone with PD to your full calendar, something's gotta give; the most likely candidate is your own regular exercise. *Stop!*

Before you go any further, take a moment to consider the following:

- Someone you love has PD and will *eventually* need help.

- You partner is managing fine with the present treatment plan. You understand that this plan can

368

last for years by monitoring the disease and using medications.

- You have a choice:

    • Project the worst as you try and control the future by making life-changing decisions right now.

    • Make reasonable plans and preparations by educating yourself about options and then living the life that's still reasonably normal.

If you elect the second option, congratulations! Plan to familiarize yourself with the information in other sections of this book, especially Parts 4 and 5. Now, about *your* body, mind, and spirit. Start by following the same guidelines we suggest in the "Exercises for the Mind and Spirit" section. Then read the Bill of Rights for the PD care partner in Chapter 19.

You don't have PD. You have a life beyond caring for this person—just as the PWP has a life beyond living with it. Mental and spiritual well being for each of you depends on maintaining normalcy as long as possible. The greatest danger is surrendering your potentially good and happy years to anxiety and depression, which can be a major factor with PD. Check out Chapter 13, where we address that concern in depth.

Books For ALL Kinds of Readers

At ReadHowYouWant we understand that one size does not fit all types of readers. Our innovative, patent pending technology allows us to design new formats to make reading easier and more enjoyable for you. This helps improve your speed of reading and your comprehension. Our EasyRead printed books have been optimized to improve word recognition, ease eye tracking by adjusting word and line spacing as well as minimizing hyphenation. Our EasyRead SuperLarge editions have been developed to make reading easier and more accessible for vision-impaired readers. We offer Braille and DAISY formats of our books and all popular E-Book formats.

We are continually introducing new formats based upon research and reader preferences. Visit our web-site to see all of our formats and learn how you can Personalize our books for yourself or as gifts. Sign up to Become A RHYW Registered Reader.

www.readhowyouwant.com

Made in the USA